Health of Black Americans from Post Reconstruction to Integration, 1871–1960

Recent Titles in
Bibliographies and Indexes in Afro-American and African Studies

Index to Afro-American Reference Resources
Rosemary M. Stevenson, compiler

A Richard Wright Bibliography:
Fifty Years of Criticism and Commentary, 1933-1982
Keneth Kinnamon, compiler, with the help of Joseph Benson, Michel Fabre,
and Craig Werner

Index of Subjects, Proverbs, and Themes in the Writings of Wole Soyinka
Greta M. K. Coger, compiler

Southern Black Creative Writers, 1829-1953: Biobibliographies
M. Marie Booth Foster, compiler

The Black Aged in the United States: A Selectively Annotated Bibliography
Lenwood G. Davis, compiler

Àshe, Traditional Religion and Healing in Sub-Saharan Africa and the
Diaspora: A Classified International Bibliography
John Gray, compiler

Black Theatre and Performance: A Pan-African Bibliography
John Gray, compiler

Health of Black Americans from Post Reconstruction to Integration, 1871–1960

An Annotated Bibliography of Contemporary Sources

Compiled by
Mitchell F. Rice
and **Woodrow Jones, Jr.**

Bibliographies and Indexes in Afro-American and African Studies, Number 26

GREENWOOD PRESS
New York • Westport, Connecticut • London

Library of Congress Cataloging-in-Publication Data

Rice, Mitchell F.
   Health of black Americans from post reconstruction to integration,
   1871-1960 : an annotated bibliography of contemporary sources /
   compiled by Mitchell F. Rice and Woodrow Jones, Jr.
      p. cm.—(Bibliographies and indexes in Afro-American and
   African studies, ISSN 0742-6925 ; no. 26)
      ISBN 0-313-26314-0 (lib. bdg. : alk. paper)
      1. Afro-Americans—Diseases—History—19th century—Abstracts.
   2. Afro-Americans—Diseases—History—20th century—Abstracts.
   3. Afro-Americans—Medical care—History—19th century—Abstracts.
   4. Afro-Americans—Medical care—History—20th century—Abstracts.
   I. Jones, Woodrow. II. Title. III. Series.
   RA448.5.N4R52   1990
   016.3621'08996073—dc20   89-78161

British Library Cataloguing in Publication Data is available.

Library of Congress Catalog Card Number: 89-78161
ISBN: 0-313-26314-0
ISSN: 0742-6925

First published in 1990

Greenwood Press, 88 Post Road West, Westport, CT 06881
An imprint of Greenwood Publishing Group, Inc.

Printed in the United States of America

∞™

The paper used in this book complies with the
Permanent Paper Standard issued by the National
Information Standards Organization (Z39.48-1984).

10 9 8 7 6 5 4 3 2 1

TO A HEALTHY
BLACK AMERICA

CONTENTS

INTRODUCTION:
BLACK HEALTH FROM
SLAVERY TO THE
MID-TWENTIETH CENTURY

The condition of blacks during the period of slavery has particular relevance for the understanding of the present condition of blacks in the American health care system. Patterns of mortality, morbidity and utilization are all rooted in the historical context in which blacks have found themselves. Since mortality is determined in part by the availability of health resources, it necessarily is impacted by economic, political, and social trends and conditions. Morbidity is also influenced by these factors but is more likely to be influenced by the availability of a regular source of care. A regular source of care allows for the exercise of preventative measures to maintain health. Social support, living and working conditions also have a direct impact on both morbidity and mortality. Despite these known causal relationships, there remains a large disparity between blacks and whites as to mortality, morbidity and utilization behaviors.

This essay reviews the literature and discusses the trends in the mortality, morbidity and the utilization behaviors of blacks from slavery to the mid-twentieth century. This discussion of the determinants of the health conditions of blacks during this period is an attempt to place the social context of black health care into perspective. Furthermore, it provides the user of the following annotated bibliography with linkages to the dominant themes of each period and a fuller understanding of the history of health care inequities in the United States.

The bibliography covers the literature published in three major time periods: (1) Post Reconstruction to the Early Twentieth Century, 1871-1919; (2) The Literature from 1920 to 1950; and (3) The Literature of the Mid-Twentieth Century, 1951-1960. In its present form we have attempted to be comprehensive but not definitive. Our focus upon the period 1870s through 1960 is deliberate because the works have not been brought together as a single unit and they are often glossed over or given cursory mention. Further, the Post-Reconstruction period serves as a good starting point because it was at this time that blacks began to leave the plantation system where a modicum of health care was provided and ventured into a social order where little or no health care was available to them. The more recent literature of the 1970s and 1980s is excluded because much of it appears in our work Black American Health: An Annotated Bibliography (Greenwood Press, 1987).

BLACK HEALTH CARE DURING SLAVERY

There are only a few accounts of black history in the United States that provide some attention to blacks health status during the slavery period. These accounts, however, do make it clear that mere survival was a preoccupation of black slaves and to some extent with slaveowners. Slaves were positively selected because of their health. Slaveowners selected young, strong blacks for transport from Africa to the United States. The weaker slaves usually succumbed to the inhumane conditions of the voyage from Africa. Due to market conditions, slave traders paid some attention to black health status after their arrival. Most slaves were bought and sold based on their physical assets and abilities, with health being a major criterion.[1]

Wealth was in part determined by the number of healthy slaves; thus, owners found it necessary to provide slaves with at least a modicum of medical care. Slaveowners even designated some slaves who had shown the ability to cure the illnesses of other slaves as doctors and "doctoresses."[2] In addition, white physicians provided medical care to slaves in order to supplement their income. Given their working conditions, slaves were a constant source of income due to their need for medical attention and care. Many black females were bought and sold based on the slave buyer's perception of their ability to bear children. With their interest in an ever growing labor supply, slaveowners saw to it that slave mothers were granted time to nurse and care for their infants. In fact, some female slaves were designated as midwives to attend to both black and white women. Children, given their value, were placed in nurseries with instructions to overseers that none of the children were to be harmed.[3]

Although census takers obtained information on births and deaths of slaves as reported to them by plantation owners and overseers, little systematic data were compiled and maintained on their health. As a result, the general mortality data collected on slaves were generally unreliable. Although the disparities between blacks and whites may not seem to be so great during the slavery era, this difference may be much larger due to underreporting of slave deaths.

HEALTH STATUS AND CONDITIONS

Sanitation and Housing

Diseases that were commonly associated with slavery were not too different from the diseases that were common for the period. Poor living conditions generally promoted infections and parasitic diseases. In addition, poor sanitation, hygiene, clothing and physical treatment were the major determinants of an individual's susceptibility to a disease.[4] The sanitation conditions in slave quarters deteriorated as the old plantation system was destroyed. Lacking the requirements of sanitation, many slaves developed health problems directly connected to poor sanitation. William F. Brunner discussed the white man's responsibility for black health care as more than the passing of sanitation laws, suggesting that unless blacks were kept in sanitary conditions, they would transmit diseases to the white community.[5]

Housing conditions in the slave quarters were far from adequate for healthy living. Usually, slaves lived and worked on farms as laborers. Their attachment to their masters was symbolized by the type of housing constructed for their use. Homes, generally, were of one room design with much overcrowding. Often more than one family would occupy one home. In such conditions personal hygiene becomes a public and not a personal concern. Poor ventilation, earthen floors, contaminated water and infested soil all contributed to an environment that was unhealthy. Poor sanitation in the slave quarters compounded the damage created by overcrowded housing. Slaves were not allowed night pots for the disposal of human waste. Instead, many slaves discharged their waste outside of their homes. The accumulation of waste products not only created the easy transferal of diseases but also the contamination of the water supply. Children playing in the slave quarter were vectors for diseases that are easily transported by hand and mouth. Epidemics in such crowded conditions could easily be traced to the slave quarters of a plantation. However, the value of a slave was tied to the health conditions within the slave quarters; thus many owners would once a year clean the waste around the slave quarters and use the accumulated waste as fertilizer.

Working Conditions
Working conditions were an important determinant of black health status. The physical treatment of slaves in the working environment varied depending on their sex and ownership. Females were not placed at the same risk due to their ability to produce more slaves and thus increase the wealth of the owner. Furthermore, females were more likely to work in capacities which were less strenuous. In contrast, males were more likely to work the fields, and therefore, more likely to suffer the hazards of prolonged exposure to weather conditions, animal bites, exposure to parasites, and contaminated water.

Slave working conditions and duties varied according to the owners' temperament. For some slaveowners the overseers' use of the whip was an important tool to enhance the speed of work. While a motivator, whippings were a health risk due to the trauma to the body and the possibilities of infections. Multiple lacerations of the skin caused the loss of blood, damage of vital organs, and permanent damage to the muscles. Frequent whippings not only decreased the value of the slave, but also decreased the body's ability to resist infections and diseases.

The literature of the period tended to focus on the health conditions of slaves. The debilitating effects of slavery and the poor health services were a central theme. The concern for the health of the slaves was not motivated by human interest, but by a concern that diseases would spread into the white population.

POST-RECONSTRUCTION HEALTH CARE

The Post-Civil War period has historically been denoted

as a period of change and frustration for blacks. The high
expectations that were experienced in the Reconstruction
period were not translated into better educational or social
realities. The defeated South was resentful of the
desegregation efforts and the new economic realities imposed
by the North. The political rights won in the South were
imposed in a manner that threatened any new social realities.
Within the atmosphere of resentment, the old slave health
care system was destroyed as the large plantations were
removed from the center of the economy of Southern states.
There was no health provider for the freed slaves, except for
the shortlived Freedmen's Bureau, and consequently their
health deteriorated. Many former slaves drifted north in the
hopes of finding a better life. Others remained as tenant
farmers to cultivate what was left of the vast estates.
     The previous value of slaves as property was a key
ingredient in their health status. In the
Post-Reconstruction period, lacking value and free, slaves
went to fellow former slaves for the delivery of health
services. However, many of these services were based on
superstitions. Frank A. Jones wrote in detail of the use of
folk remedies to drive out diseases. The use of "bug tea,"
"magnolia blossom" and "a live frog" are examples of folk
remedies suggested by these providers.[6] Former slaves who
had medical training on larger plantations were in much
demand for the provision of services. Unfortunately, the few
black doctors that were available were located in larger
communites and in Northern states. The lack of adequate
providers resulted in many blacks traveling to small towns,
where they sought services from white physicians. However,
the rise of medical science meant that blacks were now more
an object of study than of treatment.
     The studies on blacks during this period were disease
specific. For example, Seale Harris observed the prevalence
of tuberculosis and attributed the condition to poor habits
and sanitary conditions, which he blamed on blacks'
"indolence and improvidence."[7] This tone only repeats Thomas
J. Mckie's earlier assessment that insanity and tuberculosis
are linked in the black race due to "an overtaxed and
overworked nervous organization unfitted by nature and
otherwise to bear the burden imposed by newly created
necessities or environment".[8] These studies reiterate a
constant theme of slavery, that of racial inferiority. In
addressing the cocaine problem among blacks, Frank A. Jones
noted that the habit leads to "acute mania" ...and is found[9]
among the lowest and most ignorant class. The theme of
racial superiority was also the rule when surgery was needed.
Many physicians felt that blacks were poor subjects for
surgery due to their tendency not to survive. Lucien Lofton
concluded that "Surgically everything is against the Negro,[10]
physically he is operable, and without peer."

Health Status and Conditions
     In the Post-Reconstruction period the prevalence of
diseases that were common to slaves increased. Poor living
condition, poor sanitation and poor hygiene were important
factors in the transmittal of many diseases. Physical
mistreatment as a causative agent was no longer a factor in
the health condition of former slaves, but their migration to

small towns and cities exposed them to new health risks. The
migration to the city put former slaves at risk to many of
the diseases associated with overcrowding. Usually, the
migration to the city resulted in settlement patterns closely
resembling those of the slave quarters. More than one family
sharing a dwelling, the lack of resources and poor diets all
affected the health status of the new migrant. H. M. Folkes
and others placed the blame for the decreasing health
standards among blacks on the return (via emancipation) of
progeny to their "more or less fatalistic parents, who,
removed from the control of intelligent direction, soon
lapsed into their African condition of irresponsibility."[11]

Poor sanitation contributed to the high incidence of
tuberculosis among the former slaves. Waste treatment
facilities and practices varied from town to town. Waste
products were still untreated and accumulated at the
outskirts of black quarters. A. G. Fort found that less than
fifty percent of the black homes had toilets of any type and
only a small percentage of black schools and black churches
had them.[12]   Sarah B. Meyers found that white homes were also
infected with diseases because of the total lack of healthy
conditions and practices among blacks who served in the homes
of whites.[13]   For this reason she advocated the improvement
of cleanliness, mode of living, and knowledge of disease
prevention among blacks.

The tone of Meyers' analysis was even more prevalent in
the writings of those authors who focused on sexually
transmitted diseases. Much of the literature on venereal
disease takes a moralistic tone. Blacks were often described
as an "unmoral people" which accounted for the high incidence
of venereal disease. S. S. Hindman argued that ninety-five
percent of the black race would contract syphilis or some
other venereal disease.[14]   A more confronting article in the
Journal of the American Medical Association by Thomas W.
Murrell argued that teaching blacks the hygienics of the
disease was hopeless, and laws must be made that related to
blacks and only blacks, similar to laws made for Indians.[15]
L. C. Allen suggested that blacks should learn to work hard,
quit "frolicking" with members of the opposite sex, and learn
to care for their sick.[16]

In order to combat the high disease rates among blacks,
a number of health promotion campaigns were carried out by
city health departments. The New York City Department of
Health in cooperation with the National League on Urban
Conditions conducted an intensive educational campaign in the
city for two weeks.[17] Noting the ignorance on health
matters, some authors urged whites to become involved with
black health care as a way of preventing the spread of
disease in the white community.[18]   Others described the
ignorance and poverty on the part of blacks and the
indifference caused by ignorance on the part of the landlords
and voters. Thus, black health care became a part of the
growing public health movement in an industrializing society.

THE WAR YEARS AND BLACK HEALTH CARE

The first World War was a turning point in the
development of the black community. The exodus from the
South and the industrialization of the Midwest were two

prominent factors in changing the conditions of black health.
Labor-induced migrations from small towns to large cities
were the norm until the late thirties. The collapsing
southern economy and the industrialization of the Midwest
were factors in the migration of blacks. The great factory
towns of the Midwest provided not only jobs but a chance for
a better life, a life which offered new roles and
expectations for a generation that was born in the
Post-Reconstruction period.

For those who remained behind, there was a return in the
social structure to the pre-Civil War South. The
institutionalization of Jim Crow laws to restrict the
acquisition of political and social power was pronounced in
the South. Consequently, the rise of the KKK and other
racist groups and the retrenchment of black groups marked the
period. Many health providers worked in segregated health
care conditions.

Black health care personnel was a particularly important
concern in the literature during this period. Given the rise
of medical science and the requirements of a medical
education, the slave midwifes and others were no longer able
to practice medicine. Although the number of black medical
students increased during the Post-Reconstruction period,
that trend had now reversed. Numa R. G. Adams discussed the
need for better undergraduate training, scholarships and
financial aid and the acceptance of black students at white
medical schools in the North.[19] He noted that the number of
black medical students declined from 510 in 1927 to 337 in
1935. Ulysses G. Mason observed that black graduates were
admitted at very few hospitals as interns.[20] Other studies
of black physicians tended to support a black physician
shortage and decline. In a study by Paul Cornely, which
compared the 1942 distribution of black physicians with the
distribution in 1932, the ratio of black physicians to the
black population was still much greater than the 1 to 750 for
all physicians.[21] When controlling for region of the
country, the South as a whole showed the lowest ratio. Since
black physicians tended to concentrate in large cities,
nearly all southern states showed ratios which were lower
than the national average.

Allied health professionals, especially nurses were also
in short supply. Before World War II there were few schools
of nursing which would admit blacks for training. Between
1941 and 1949, 325 additional schools opened doors to
blacks.[22] Following the war the National Nursing Council
made an effort to appeal to black youth to consider the
opportunities that existed due to the expansion of health
services to a larger section of the population. Still, among
the 1,300 accredited nursing schools in 1946, only 28 were
for blacks.[23]

Like the shortage of physicians, the nursing shortage
was more severely felt in rural settings. Many southern
small cities were without adequate nursing support to
supplement health care needs. Better pay and benefits were
available in the larger cities. In 1944 there were some 124
black hospitals in the country[24] in which the demand for
black nurses was quite high. However, in white hospitals,
black nurses were ostracized by others in the profession as
not being capable of performing their tasks. Furthermore,

hospital administrators were likely to hire young black nurses at lower wages.

Health Status and Conditions

Between the two world wars the health conditions of black men who were in the service improved. These men were better treated and were more conscious of venereal diseases, dentistry, and surgical care. Throughout their military experience, they were provided with a regular source of care and socialization to the use of medical services. However, the general health conditions of the rest of the black population did not improve. The depression of the 1930's created a great migration Northward from the rural South. The difference in environment had real impact on the availability of care and the health of the population. Walter R. Chivers cited numerous studies of the effects of migration on tuberculosis, syphilis, and psychopathic sequelae.[25] The high incidence of these diseases was attributed to the change in living conditions. Housing in large black ghettoes in urban areas was frequently worse than in rural areas. However, the increased availability of medical services and the means of evaluating mortality and morbidity may also account for the increased number of cases reported or discovered.

The psychological stresses of the migration and the lack of recreational outlets led to increasing numbers of mental disorders among blacks. Environmental and social stress increased not only crime but also suicide rates. Walter A. Adams argued that the unacceptability of mental disorders to most blacks prevented effective treatment for stress related disorders. Further, he argued that therapists "who accept Negro patients must examine with considerable care their attitudes and feelings toward race, and they should also possess a knowledge of the structure and cultural background of the Negro social group."[26]

The change in labor force participation also produced stress in migrants. A study of black factory workers over age twenty in Cincinnati conducted by Floyd P. Allen found only one of the 1,000 men examined was free of any physical defects.[27] Most of the men had significant cardiovascular abnormalities and over two hundred had hypertension. The outstanding communicable disease among them was tuberculosis. These findings are not surprising given the typical industrial city, where blacks were quartered along railroad tracks or dirty streams.

Tuberculosis was the dominant health concern in the North as well as the South. James A. Crabtree's study of blacks in a small Tennessee city found that those households where tuberculosis was discovered were more crowded, had larger families, had lower milk consumption, and were dirty and untidy.[28] Louis I. Dublin argued that blacks who escaped tuberculosis infection during childhood were more likely to suffer in adult life from rapidly fatal tuberculosis with the characteristics of the first infection of white children.[29] Elaine Ellis's writing in Crisis summarized that "because conditions were even worse in the South, southern blacks have the highest tuberculosis mortality in America."[30]

The moral tones of the previous period against the epidemic of syphilis were replaced with scientific studies of

the epidemic. H. H. Hazen's study provided data suggesting
that blacks were more likely than whites to suffer from
syphilis and were more likely to go untreated until the late
stages of the disease.[31]   Data in the study suggested that
black women suffered at higher rates than white women. James
A. Crabtree and others' study of rural Tennessee estimated an
annual morbidity rate from syphilis of approximately 4,333
per 100,000.[32]   Some states made direct efforts at health
promotion through the use of mobile clinics and educational
campaigns. However, the lack of public health facilities to
provide treatment services and follow-up prevented a decline
in mortality.
    A new issue of concern in the literature was the rising
infant mortality rate among blacks. Elizabeth C. Tandy, a
Senior Statistician for the Children's Bureau of the U.S.
Department of Labor, found that only 20 percent of black
births in the rural South were attended by physicians.
Southern states exhibited high infant mortality rates as a
whole, but black infant mortality rates were 80.2 per 1000
live births in the rural South and 109.3 per 1000 live births
in the urban South.[33]   In every category of disease, black
infants had a higher mortality rate than white infants. The
lack of birth control, poor maternal education and poverty
were all factors in these high rates. In a study of maternal
attitudes toward birth control, Preston Valien and others
noted that many of the mothers had reservations centered
around the sinfulness of birth control.[34]   However, education
and urbanization tended to reduce the fear of birth control.
Thus, ignorance, as well as poor hygienic surroundings,
seriously influenced the maternity situation in an adverse
manner.

MID-TWENTIETH CENTURY BLACK HEALTH CARE

    The impact of the Korean War was similar to World War II
in the black community. The mobilization for war required
the desegregation of the work force. For the first time
women and minorities were involved in the workforce in large
numbers. Efforts to equalize benefits and pay were the
keynotes of the administration. The resulting efforts
induced migration to cities with war-related industries. The
aftermath of the war years can be seen in the efforts to
desegregate schooling and promote civil rights in health care
as well as in society in general. The war years and the
growing demand for civil rights created a greater social
consciousness within the medical profession. The old slave
health care system had ended with the movement to desegregate
the delivery of medical services in the society. Black
nurses and doctors were finally admitted to several medical
societies. Furthermore, black nurses were now being hired by
white hospitals in the North. However, in the South these
changes were very slow in coming and the pattern of
segregated health care remained.
    W. M. Cobb, a longtime editor of The Journal of the
National Medical Association, noted in Hospital Management
that only 2 percent of physicians in the United States were
black in 1959.[35]   When trying to join hospital staffs, the
black physician encountered the same problems which hindered
his entering the medical profession. Because of these

barriers, many black physicians opened private clinics which served the needs of the black poor. Black nurses were equally underrepresented in the nursing population and the hiring of black nurses in white hospitals after the war had an impact on black hospitals and clinics. Rhoda L. Goldstein's study of black staff nurses at white hospitals found that the largest obstacle for the black nurse involved acceptance on the part of both her colleagues and patients.[36] Black nurses met with attitudes of indifference, prejudice and disdain upon their arrival and they faced limited opportunities for promotion and authority.

The call for national health insurance was symbolic of the new demands being placed on the health care system. Oscar R. Ewing, Federal Security Administrator, called for a national health insurance program with a nondiscriminatory clause to improve black health status.[37]   Taft Raines also argued that public funds should not be spent on institutions which practiced discrimination and that Blue Cross should not approve hospitals that practiced discrimination.[38]

Health Status and Problems

Given the excellent health care of blacks who had served during the war, there now was a bifurcation of the health status and problems in the black community. While black members of the military were in excellent health, the rest of the black community was not. A detailed analysis of mortality by Maryland Pennell and Mary Grover in 1951 found seven causes of death in which blacks and whites differed.[39] There was a higher mortality rate for blacks from tuberculosis, nephritis, influenza and pneumonia, intracranial lesions of vascular origins, diseases of the heart, syphilis, and homicide.

The issue of infant mortality did not wane in the literature of the period. Studies such as Jose Fontanilla and George Anderson's 1955 report on the incidence of ectopic pregnancies indicated a higher incidence among blacks.[40]   The cause of this higher incidence was attributed to pelvic inflammatory disease, specifically gonorrhea. Maternal deaths due to ectopic pregnancies were also higher in black women. Eleanor Payton, E. Perry Crump and Carrell P. Horton, writing a few years later, also noted that pregnant black women were deficient in recommended nutrients. Economic circumstances, food dislikes, and a lack of knowledge concerning nutritional needs explained the omission of vital nutrients in diets.[41]

A new focus in the literature was the mental health of blacks. The postwar period was marked by a reversal of the expectations generated by the war. As the soldiers returned, they encountered old patterns of behavior, including denial of rights, prejudice, and economic discrimination. Blacks in the postwar period were again experiencing the kind of stress experienced by the post migration generation. The literature examining the impact of segregation on the mental health of blacks tended to focus on senile psychosis, arteriosclerotic dementia and schizophrenia. David C. Wilson and others found that blacks in Virginia, whose admission rates were higher than whites, were more likely to be diagnosed with these conditions. Between 1914 and 1955 the white admission ratio increased by 113 points; the black ratio increased by 343

points. The admission ratio per 100,000 black population had
more than doubled in the forty-year period.[42]
     The abuse of alcohol became a characteristic of the
inner city black population. Benjamin Malzberg focused on
the frequency of alcoholic psychoses among black first
admissions to hospitals for mental disease in the state of
New York. He argued that alcohol plays a more significant
role in the frequency of these psychoses for blacks than for
whites.[43]   R. A. Schermerhorn argued that many of the
disorders experienced by blacks were due to the lower class
nature of the population, the resulting strain of
unemployment and feelings of inferiority.[44]   In addition,
segregation and uncertainty of cultural change resulted in
increasing rate of admission of black clients in state mental
hospitals.
     Sexually transmitted diseases were still a major focus
of public health efforts during the mid-century period. The
results of several long-term studies of black syphilitic men
were being reported in the literature. Sidney Olansky and
others' study of 431 men found that 40.8 percent died by the
end of the study. The death rate ranged from 18 percent for
those with syphilis of ten years of less to 96 percent among
those who had syphilis forty years or more.[45]   The famous
Tuskegee study also showed that there was a higher rate of
cardiac problems in the syphilitic group which suggests that
syphilis could predispose a patient to heart problems.[46]
Many patients were allowed to die in order to determine the
severity of the disease. Cooperation in this study was
obtained by the offering of free burial assistance and other
inducements. Eunice Rivers and others argued that the
experience of this project was beneficial as guidance for
further long-term studies. Some factors for program success
include being aware of incentives that produce maximum
cooperation, keep strong rapport between patient and
physician, and awareness that changes in key personnel could
have an impact on the entire project.[47]
     In sum, the mid-twentieth century literature on black
health care did not differ from that of the war period.
Gross disparities in the health care system were evidenced
for northern and southern black populations. Consequently,
the medical care system, unable to meet these new demands,
was poised for transformation at the end of this period.
Unfortunately for many blacks these changes would be
implemented too late to counteract the effects of years of
neglect.

CONCLUSION

     Over the past 100 years the health care industry in the
United States has become an important sector of the economy.
It no longer just provides medical services; it is a
multi-billion dollar industry. Despite the advances in the
reduction of mortality and morbidity, there are still
disparities between blacks and whites on every measure of
illness and death. These disparities have existed over time
and have become a consistent reality for each new cohort of
black citizens. Governmental programs and policies were
implemented rather late in the black community. Many federal
programs were so underfunded and poorly implemented that

their impact has been sporadic and misdirected. In addition, the failure to design programs that target blacks as a special group and follow-up with broad social changes has resulted in further decline of the health of the black population. Health care reflects the general conditions of people within the population. It reflects the matrix of social, economic and political factors that segment a society. The history of black health care also reflects the general conditions of blacks within the general population. Clearly, what can be learned from this historical analysis are some of the causal factors that created and still maintain the disparities between black and white health care.

There is support within this literature of three explanations for the health disparities between blacks and whites. First, institutional racism as an explanation focuses on the exclusion of blacks from the medical care system. Historically, the period from the end of slavery to the second World War provides evidence of exclusion from medical services in most Southern states. During slavery blacks were given better primary care only because of their property value. Even in the North blacks received poor health care as a result of biases in public facilities and the lack of medical personnel.

The second explanation centers on the economic inequality in the society which prevented blacks from obtaining health care. Poverty from the Post-Reconstruction period forward was an important factor in preventing the attainment of adequate health insurance. Lacking skills, adequate housing and education, the early black migrant to the city was not equipped to attain the resources necessary to purchase health care. Furthermore, there were few black hospitals and even fewer black doctors to provide health services before the second World War.

The final explanation focuses on access barriers within the medical care system. Attitudes and perceptions of health and health behaviors are bound by traditions and culture. The folk beliefs of blacks about health are grounded in diverse socialization and religious experiences. In the slave and Post-Reconstruction period, there was a reliance on folk remedies and not medical practice. On the other hand, the viewpoint of the provider is another access barrier.

A consistent theme in all periods of the literature studied was a negative image of blacks by white providers, which prevented black patients from developing trust in white providers and modern medical practice. In sum, these causal factors contribute to a partial explanation of the development of a historical pattern of inequity. Each explanation can be directly linked to the failure of government to move aggressively in terms of social equality and protection of the political rights of blacks in the larger community. This failure underlies many of the excessive deaths of blacks compared to whites. Unfortunately, until there is some change in policy direction, the next hundred years will be only a variation of the past.

The annotated bibliography that follows resulted from the work of many individuals. We would like to thank our graduate assistants and a number of graduate students who performed uncounted hours of library research. We would like to thank Gayla Chapman for her excellent secretarial assistance. For errors of omission or commission, we accept full responsibility.

NOTES

[1] See Martha Carolyn Mitchell, "Health and the Medical Profession in the Lower South, 1845-1860." Journal of Southern History 10 (1944): 424-446.

[2] See Ibid. and Weymouth T. Jordan, "Plantation Medicine in the Old South." Alabama Review 3 (1950): 83-107.

[3] See W. D. Postell, "Birth and Mortality Among Slave Infants on Southern Plantations." Pediatrics 10 (November 1952): 538-541.

[4] See Horace W. Clark, "The Health of the Negroes in the South: The Great Cause of Mortality Among Them: The Causes and Remedies." Sanitarian 18 (1887): 502-518; and Felice Swados, "Negro Health on the Antebellum Plantation." Bulletin of the History of Medicine 10 (1941): 460-472.

[5] William F. Brunner, "The Negro Health Problem in Southern Cities," American Journal of Public Health 5 (March 1915): 183-190.

[6] Frank A. Jones, "Some Superstitions Among the Southern Negroes," Journal of the American Medical Association 50 (15) (April 11, 1908): 1207.

[7] Seale Harris, "Tuberculosis in the Negro." Journal of the American Medical Association 41 (14) (October 3, 1903): 834-838.

[8] Thomas J. Mckie, "A Brief History of Insanity and Tuberculosis in the Southern Negro." Journal of the American Medical Association 28 (12) (March 20, 1897): 537-538.

[9] Frank A. Jones, "Cocain Habit Among the Negroes." Journal of the American Medical Association 35 (3) (July 21, 1900): 175.

[10] Lucien Lofton, "The Negro as a Surgical Subject." New Orleans Medical and Surgical Journal 54 (February 1902): 530-533.

[11] H. M. Folkes, "The Negro as a Health Problem." Journal of the American Medical Association (15) (October 8, 1910): 1246-1247.

[12] A. G. Fort, "The Negro Health Problem in Rural Communities." American Journal of Public Health 5 (March 1915): 183-190.

[13] Sarah B. Meyers, "The Negro Problem as it Appears to a Public Health Nurse." The American Journal of Nursing 19 (1918): 278-281.

14 S. S. Hindman, "Syphilis Among Insane Negroes." American Journal of Public Health 5 (3) (1915): 213-224.

15 Thomas W. Murrell, "Syphilis and the American Negro." Journal of the American Medical Association 54 (11) (March 12, 1910): 846-849.

16 L. C. Allen, "The Negro Health Problem." American Journal of Public Health 5 (1915): 194-203.

17 "Health Campaign Among Negroes." American Journal of Public Health 7 (Summer 1917): 510.

18 See, for example, C. E. Terry, "The Negro: His Relation to Public Health in the South." American Journal of Public Health 3 (1913): 300-310 and M. L. Graves, "Practical Remedial Measures for the Improvement of Hygienic Conditions in the South." American Journal of Public Health 5 (March 1915): 191-193.

19 Numa P. G. Adams, "Sources of Supply of Negro Health Personnel: Physicians." Journal of Negro Education 6 (1937): 468-476.

20 Ulysses G. Mason, "Problems Incidental to Negro Staff Training in Hospitals." Hospitals 3 (March 1944): 71-72.

21 Paul Cornely, "Segregation and Discrimination in Medical Care in the United States." American Journal of Public Health 46 (September 1956): 1074-1081.

22 See Estelle Massey Osborne, "Status and Contribution of the Negro Nurse." The Journal of Negro Education 18 (Summer 1949): 364-369.

23 See Estelle Massey Riddle, "The Nurse Shortage - A Concern of the Negro Public." Opportunity 25 (January 1947): 22-23.

24 E. H. Bradley, "Health, Hospitals and the Negro." Modern Hospital 65 (August 1945): 43-44.

25 Walter R. Chivers, "Northward Migration and the Health of Negroes." The Journal of Negro Education 8 (January 1939): 34-43.

26 Walter A. Adams, "The Negro Patient in Psychiatric Treatment," American Journal of Orthopsychiatry 20 (2) (April 1950): 305-310.

27 Floyd P. Allen, "Physical Impairment Among One Thousand Negro Workers." American Journal of Public Health 22 (June 1932): 579-586.

28 James A. Crabtree, "Tuberculosis Studies in Tennessee: Tuberculosis in the Negro as Related to Certain Conditions of Environment." Journal of the American Medical Association 101 (10) (September 2, 1933): 756-761.

[29] Louis I. Dublin, "The Epidemiology of Tuberculosis of Negroes," American Journal of Public Health 21 (March 1931): 290-291.

[30] Elaine Ellis, "Tuberculosis Among Negroes." Crisis 46 (4) (April 1939): 112, 125.

[31] H. H. Hazen, "A Leading Cause of Death Among Negroes: Syphilis." Journal of Negro Education 6 (1937): 310-321.

[32] James A. Crabtree et al, "Syphilis in a Rural Negro Population in Tennessee," American Journal of Public Health 22 (February 1932): 157-164.

[33] Elizabeth C. Tandy, "Infant and Maternal Mortality Among Negroes." Journal of Negro Education 6 (1937): 322-349.

[34] Preston Valien et al, "Attitudes of the Negro Mother Toward Birth Control." American Journal of Sociology 55 (November 1949): 279-283.

[35] W. M. Cobb, "The Negro Physician and Hospital Staffs." Hospital Management (March 1960): 22-24.

[36] Rhoda L. Goldstein, "Negro Nurses in Hospitals." American Journal of Nursing 60 (February 1960): 215-217.

[37] Oscar R. Ewing, "Facing the Facts of Negro Health." Crisis 59 (4) (April 1952): 217-222, 261-262.

[38] Taft Raines, "Barriers to Community Health." Modern Hospital 79 (August 1952): 71-73.

[39] Maryland Pennell and Mary Grover, "Urban and Rural Mortality from Selected Causes in the North and South." Public Health Reports 66 (10) (March 9, 1951): 295-305.

[40] Jose Fontanilla and George Anderson, "Further Studies of the Racial Incidence and Mortality from Ectopic Pregnancy." American Journal of Obstetrics and Gynecology 70 (2) (August 1955): 312-319.

[41] Eleanor Payton, E. Perry Crump and Carrell P. Horton, "Growth and Development." Journal of the American Dietetic Association 37 (August 1960): 129-136.

[42] David C. Wilson et al, "The Effect of Culture on the Negro Race in Virginia, as Indicated by a Study of State Hospital Admissions." American Journal of Psychiatry 114 (July 1957): 25-32.

[43] Benjamin Malzberg, "Use of Alcohol Among White and Negro Mental Patients." Quarterly Journal of Studies on Alcohol 16 (1955): 668-674.

[44] R. A. Schermerhorn, "Psychiatric Disorders Among Negroes: A Sociological Note." American Journal of Psychiatry (May 1956): 878-882.

[45] Sidney Olansky et al, "Untreated Syphilis in the Male Negro." Archives of Dermatology 73 (May 1956): 516-529.

[46] See Sidney Olansky et al, "Untreated Syphilis in the Negro Male." Journal of Chronic Disease 4 (2) (August 1956): 177-185.

[47] Eunice Rivers et al, "Twenty Years of Followup Experience in a Long-Range Medical Study." Public Health Reports 68 (4) (April 1953): 391-395.

1

POST RECONSTRUCTION TO THE EARLY TWENTIETH CENTURY, 1871–1919

001. Abel, J. J. and Davis, W. S. "On The Pigment of the Negro's Skin and Hair," The Journal of Experimental Medicine 1 (3) (July 1896)): 361-400.

Experiments were done on the pigments of the epidermis of the dark-skinned body tissues and hair which were little-known to the scientist. Details the methods of the pigment experiment of the black subject and some earlier work done in the same field. Found that the pigmentary granules on blacks were insoluble in dilute alkalines, dilute hydrochloric acid (hot or cold), alcohol, and other organic solvents. The experiments showed that the pigment was derived from the proteins of parenchymatous juices rather than from a derivative of hemoglobin. The total quantity of soluble pigment in the skin of the black of average size was found to weigh about 1 gram, the weight of the pigmentary granules was about 3.3 grams, and contained 65 percent water and 5 percent mineral constituents in natural state in the epidermis.

002. Afflect, Thomas. "On the Hygiene of Cotton Plantations and the Management of Negro Slaves," Southern Medical Reports 2 (1890): 430-435.

The principal causes of sickness among slaves on Southern plantations are the use of spring, well, creek, or bayou water. However, the slaves are generally well cared for. They are given plenty to eat. Their diet usually consists of well cooked pork. Every now and then fish and mollasses is included. Slave homes are very well built. Each home is usually from 16 to 20 feet square and has a porch or an additional bedroom. Slaves are dressed comfortably in strong woolen jeans and given two round about shirts. As for work, it is quite uniform. The slave follows the same ritual every day. At daybreak they are awakened by bells or horns. The mothers gather children at nurseries and work commences. They carry their meals to the fields and are given adequate breaks for eating. They usually stop around sundown so as to get to bed early. Slave children are managed by the older slave women who are

unable to work. They usually die at a rate of 2 to 1 as
compared to white children. The slave mother is allowed
to come in every 3 to 4 hours to breast feed the child
until the age of 9 months. However, most children die
from infections given them by other filthy slave
children. Of those born, over half will die before the
age of one.

003. Allen, L. C. "The Negro Health Problem," American
Journal of Public Health 5 (1915): 194-203.

The author, a medical doctor from Hoschton, Georgia,
chief interest in black health care is to prevent the
spread of communicable diseases from blacks to whites.
Although some data are presented , the greatest part of
the article attempts to urge whites to help blacks live
healthier, cleaner, and more moral lives. The tone of
the article is much in keeping with the
turn-of-the-century literature that is characterized by
appeals to morality. According to the author, blacks
must be taught to stop their bad habits. Many diseases
in the black community can be prevented if blacks will
clean up after themselves and stop neglecting their
children. Blacks should learn to work hard, quit
"frolicking" with members of the opposite sex, and learn
to care for their sick. Points out that blacks suffer
from nutritional deficiencies because of lack of
financial resources. His only solution lies in
education. Blacks must be taught methods of preventing
diseases as well as "book learning" in the public
schools. In addition, public school education should
teach religiosity and the benefits of initiative and
hard work.

004. "A Long-Haired Colored Woman," Journal of the American
Medical Association 26 (2) (January 11, 1896): 94.

In Leslie's Weekly for January 2nd is an account, with
illustration, of the "only living long-haired negress,"
Mary Garrison, Holly Springs, Mississippi, a true negro,
black with kinky hair, age 48. When she was 30, a
change took place in her hair following an attack of
fever. After convalescence, her short kinky hair began
to grow rapidly. In one year it grew from 3 inches to 3
feet, thickening as it grew. A few years later it fell
below her knees and turned color to white. It remained
white until two years ago and is now black. It
continued to grow and now measures 11 feet. Prominent
physicians have examined her head and hair and are
disposed to think that the spell of fever produced the
unnatural growth. Nancy is a living curiosity, visited
by hundreds who handled her massive braids before they
believe the truth.

005. "An Inherited Anomaly," Journal of the American Medical
Association 60 (9) (March 1, 1913):673-674.

A comment on a family of blacks which have a spotted
skin condition. "The 'piebald' condition of the skin,

which is spotted with white in a fairly definite pattern not unlike that of certain domesticated animals, made its appearance as a mutation or sport in a negro family of the Southern United States about sixty years ago." Notes that this family has been studied by students of heredity and that this trait behaves as a simple mendelian dominant character. Speculates that if by chance two spotted individuals of this race should marry then a new type of individual would be produced and would transmit the unique character in all its germ cells.

006. Barber, J. Max. "The Philadelphia Dentist," Crisis 7 (4) (February 1914):179-181.

Discusses the life of black dentists in Philadelphia and argues that the black dentist, like other Negro professionals, is not patronized by his own race. "Here, as all over the country, there were many colored people who did not, at first, patronize the colored dentist. This is the experience of all men of color in the professions." However, emphasizes that the black professional man soon dispels doubts of his abilities. There are plenty of black dentists in Philadelphia in 1914. These dentists handle an average of seventy-five patients a day.

007. Barrier, James M. "Tuberculosis Among Our Negroes in Louisiana," Louisiana State Medical Society: Transactions 23 (1902): 130-138.

Observes that "The Negro was liberated from slavery, given political freedom, public schools open to him,... and yet there is still a negro problem which confronts us [whites]; that is the sanitary condition of the race." Presents data on white versus black tuberculosis cases in Louisiana circa 1900. "Of 253 cases of Tb. in negroes over twelve months, 70% died and only 15% improved. Compares this to 175 cases amongst whites wherein 33.3% improved and only 40% died." Argues that sanitary conditions in black communities are the cause of the 70% death rate in black tuberculosis patients.

008. Boas, Ernst Philip. "The Relative Prevalence of Syphilis Among Negroes and Whites," Social Hygiene 1 (September 1914-1915): 410-516.

Draws attention to the shortage of valid data on the incidence of syphilis among blacks based upon numerous statistical studies on the subject. Many of the investigations were done in hospitals, dispensaries and insane asylums, such as Bellevue Hospital in New York City, 1915, Johns Hopkins Hospital (1892 to 1911), Boston Psychopathic Hospital and the Georgia State Sanitarium. Based upon these findings and the numerous factors considered, contends that these data represent only rough estimates of the prevalence of the disease and infers that these statistics are valuable in indicating the relative incidence of syphilis among

blacks and Caucasians. The data is not accurate as to
the percentage of blacks who are syphilitic. Points out
that inadequate data is characteristic of American
institutions. Furthermore, observations such as 75
percent of the black population have syphilis are
totally exaggerated and point to a low incidence of
syphilis. Questions whether blacks seek medical
attention in medical facilities and institutions as
often as do Caucasians and suggests that because
syphilis could be latent in a person without showing
symptoms or clinical signs over a period of time, that
cases are overlooked many times in hospitals. Moreover,
positive reactions to the Wassermann test which is
included as a basic criterion is not a 100 percent
certainty. Oftentimes, when a patient is admitted for
heart disease, cases are classified in the death
statistics as cardiac arrest instead of death from
syphilitic affection.

009. Boas, Frank. "The Real Race Problem," Crisis 1 (2)
(November 1911):22-25.

Presents the results of scientific investigations which
prove that the black is not inferior to the white.
Considers the size of the brain of blacks in comparison
with whites and points out that other researchers have
concluded that the brain of blacks is smaller than that
of whites. Also emphasizes that studies of the size of
the brains of great men, criminals, and normal
individuals have demonstrated that the relation between
mental ability and brain-weight is rather remote, and
"that we are not by any means justified in concluding
that the larger brain is always the more efficient tool
for mental achievement." Concludes that "the whole
anatomical and physiological comparisons of the Negro
and the white race may be summed up in the statement
that certain differences between the two races are so
fundamental that they seem to form two quite distinct
groups of the human species."

010. Brunner, William F. "The Negro Health Problem in
Southern Cities," American Journal of Public Health 5 (March
1915):183-90.

Discusses the white man's responsibility for black
health care. Argues that unless blacks are kept in
sanitary (not necessarily health) conditions, they can
transmit diseases to the white community. Several
reasons why whites must take responsibility for black
health care are: 1) there are more blacks than the white
population could support; 2) blacks live in such a
fashion that all rules of sanitation are broken; and 3)
blacks can not help themselves. Therefore, merely
passing sanitary laws is not effective.

011. Burr, Charles W. "Paralysis Agitans in Negroes,"
Journal of the American Medical Association 60 (1) (January
4, 1913):43-44.

Reports a case of paralysis agitans in a black male
because it is the only case to be documented in a black.
Presents the symptoms and justifications for the
diagnosis. Discusses some reasons that certain diseases
have not been found in different races and the
possibility of racial immunity, but also acknowledges
the possibility of the absence of the cause of some
diseases in the races. With paralysis agitans no
explanation is provided. Also notes that paralysis
agitans may not be a nervous disease but may be a
muscular one and that the rarity of its occurrence in
blacks may be due to muscular development.

012. Cartwright, Samuel. "The Diseases and Physical
Peculiarities of the Negro Race," New Orleans Surgical and
Medical Journal (1871): 421-427.

There are certain anatomical peculiarities that separate
blacks from whites. Medical remedies that would cure a
white man could very well kill a black. It is therefore
the duty of medicine and those who practice it to define
these differences so that it may aid not only whites,
but blacks as well. Because of these differences, many
white physicians have been unable to treat the diseases
associated with the black race. There is an unpopular
notion held by Northern physicians that the black is a
white man who through some genetic mutation turn out
black. However, the black's color is not by accident.
It can be explained in his inferiority to white men.
Therefore, medical education for the treatment of blacks
should be separate from that of whites. There is
nothing to prevent young white physicians from
adequately treating the diseases of the black race if
they are made aware of the anatomical and physiological
differences.

013. "The Colored Race in Life Assurance," Journal of the
American Medical Association 30 (5) (April 9, 1898):874.

A summary of a report issued by Atlanta University which
presents data on the leading causes of death among
blacks with the prevailing causes being scrofula,
infantile and pulmonary diseases. Also discusses the
experience of two life insurance companies, Prudential
and Sun Life. Both companies write insurance on a
discriminating basis due to the difference in mortality
rates.

014. "Conference on Betterment of Hygienic Conditions Among
Negroes," American Journal of Public Health 4 (Summer
1914):467.

A summary of a conference on the betterment of black
health held in New Orleans. The purpose of the meeting
was to agree on practical measures for the ultimate and
immediate betterment of blacks. The meeting was
attended by both black and white leaders in the health
field who recognized sanitation as a major problem in

the black community. Reports the resolutions and
guidelines adopted by the conference.

015.   Conrad, Horace W. "The Health of the Negroes in the
South: The Great Cause of Mortality Among Them; The Causes
and Remedies," Sanitarian 18 (1887): 502-518.

There have been reports to suggest that since the
emancipation of slaves, they have become much more
susceptable to disease and thus mortality from disease.
Prior to this time, the Master was responsible for the
care of his slaves. They provided adequate housing,
clothing, diets, and sanitation. As a result, they were
almost totally immune from disease. However, in order
to understand the true nature of the problem, one must
consider the nature of blacks' dwellings now in regard
to their dwellings prior to freedom. Data reveal that
blacks residing in Northern cities are much more likely
to contract diseases and die than those in the South.
The two greatest diseases contributing to black
mortality are pneumonia and consumption. These diseases
are directly proportioned according to the condition of
black housing. Most blacks live in under ventilated and
poorly sanitated homes. Their homes lack windows to
provide the necessary ventilation and sunlight necessary
to maintain a proper health status. They drink water
that is often contaminated and relieve themselves in
close proximity to their homes. Their diseases are
augmented by improper diets. Blacks tend to be red meat
eaters. Physicians now know that red meat in large
quantities can be very unhealthful. The prevalence of
certain diseases such as scrofula is due to a very high
intake of red meat, without a sufficient intake of
vegetables. Medical history shows that blacks while in
Africa had no known cases of this disease because their
diet consisted mainly of vegetables. Overall,
unwholesome diets have much to do with mortality among
adult blacks and infants. Another problem with
mortality in black infants is lack of adequate medical
attention. They are often treated by root doctors and
unskilled midwives. The remedy is thus to improve black
dwellings and educate caretakers as to new methods of
safer medical delivery. Intelligent blacks must lead
the way and provide for the more abundant and ignorant
blacks.

016.   Cowgill, Warwick. "Why the Negro Does Not Suffer From
Trachoma," Journal of the American Medical Association 34
(17) (February 17, 1900):399-400.

Challenges the view that blacks do not get trachoma
because they are immune to the disease. Argues that
trachoma is a contagious disease and that it is not
common among blacks because they do not come into
contact with the disease. Notes that the prevalence of
the disease is among poor whites and that the disease is
spread by the use of a single towel by all members of
the household. Points out that blacks and poor whites

have little, if any immediate contact, therefore, blacks
do not contract the disease from the whites.

017. "Do Negroes Recover from Phithisis?" Journal of the
American Medical Association 40 (22) (May 20, 1903):1520.

The question was asked by Dr. Francis Crosson in the
above issue. The information was requested from
physicians residing in the South who had considerable
numbers of cases of pulmonary tuberculosis among the
African race, if they knew any who recovered. The
responses appeared in the June 13, 1903 issue Volume 40
(24), pages 1061-1662. Dr. John Ashcroft of Atlanta,
Georgia had 15 years experience and could not recall a
single case in which treatment made the slightest
impression. Dr. E. A. Cobleigh of Chattanooga,
Tennessee writes that he doesn't recall a single case to
recover. He writes "that when a negro becomes visibly
affected with pulmonary phithisis his doom is already
practically sealed." Dr. E. D. Bondurant of Mobile,
Alabama writes that the mortality is greater in the
black race than in the white race and that the disease
runs a more rapidly fatal course in blacks. Reports
that he knows two cases to have recovered. Dr. W. H.
Barr, Agricultural College Mississippi, writes he knows
of only one case to recover in 28 years. He also feels
that the habit of sleeping with their heads covered adds
much to the succumbing to tuberculosis.

018. Ellett, E. C. "Diseases of the Ear, Nose, and Throat
in the Negro," Journal of the American Medical Association 32
(23) (December 2, 1899):1419-1420.

A summary of a paper presented to the Tri-State Medical
Association of Mississippi, Arkansas and Tennessee,
November, 1899. Concludes that: 1) blacks enjoy a
singular immunity from catarrhal inflammation, 2) blacks
are prone to Tuberculosis and syphilis, 3) blacks afford
ample opportunity to study the natural history of
disease with treatment. The author notes a number of
diseases of the eye and points out whether he has seen
them frequently, commonly or rarely.

019. Folkes, H. M. "The Negro as a Health Problem," Journal
of the American Medical Association (15) (October 8,
1910):1246-1247.

A "born and bred Southerner" the author discusses
several health-related problems characteristic of the
"Negro race" which he has encountered in his practice in
Biloxi, Mississippi. Describing the black race as
fatalistic, the author places blame for the decreasing
health standards among blacks on the return (via
emancipation) of progeny to their "more or less
fatalistic parents, who removed from the control of
intelligent direction, soon lapsed into their African
condition of irresponsibility." Also points out that
the black race has inherent immunities to diseases such
as malaria, typhoid, intestinal diseases, tonsillitis,

mumps, influenza and yellow fever. Notes the high
incidence of tuberculosis which is attributed to the
unsanitary habits of blacks such as spitting. Describes
blacks as an "unmoral people" which accounts for the
high incidence of disease, especially venereal diseases.
Concludes by expressing concern that diseases carried
and spread by blacks may infiltrate the white race
through the practice of miscegenation begun in the
North. Against this practice observes that "if decided
steps are not taken against this curse by the white
people of that part of the country, they are creating
for their descendants a Frankenstein monster indeed."

020. Fort, A. G. "The Negro Health Problem in Rural
Communities," American Journal of Public Health 5 (March
1915):183-190.

Identifies the cause of the black health problem in
rural communities as ignorance and poverty on the part
of blacks and indifference caused by ignorance on the
part of the landlords and voters. Sanitary laws are a
cause of disease among blacks. Less than fifty percent
of black homes have toilets of any type and only a small
percentage of black schools and black churches.
Concludes that knowledge is the key to stamping out all
preventable diseases.

021. Fox, Howard. "A Case of Annular Papular Syphilis in a
Negress," Journal of the American Medical Association 60 (19)
(March 10, 1913):1420-1421.

Notes that while some diseases are well known to be
characteristic of blacks, annular syphilis, while not as
well known, is also characteristic of the race.
Discusses the diagnostic criteria and a case (including
a picture of the individual with the characteristic
eruptions).

022. "Graduate Medical Fellowships for Negroes," Journal of
the American Medical Association 73 (12) (September 20,
1919):923.

This note in the Medical News Section states, "Mr.
Julius Rosenwald, Chicago, is offering six fellowships
to Negro graduates in medicine by which they may pursue
advanced studies in the fundamental medical sciences
under favorable conditions. Each stipend pays $1,200 to
cover transportation, laboratory, tuition fees, books
and living expenses."

023. Graves, M. L. "Practical Remedial Measures for the
Improvement of Hygenic Conditions in the South," American
Journal of Public Health 5 (March 1915):191-93.

Notes that the average life of blacks is about 35 years.
Estimates that some 450,000 blacks in the South are
seriously ill all the time and loose 18 days per year
from work. Some solutions suggested include: 1) the
establishment of a national department of Public Health

in the United States Government; 2) private philanthropy to finance a commission of research; 3) the enlargement and encouragement of the educational efforts of the institutions of the colored people; 4) the inauguration of public health and preventive medicine courses of instruction; 5) organization of efficient state, county, and municipal health deparments; 6) collaboration with churches and social welfare workers; 7) public schools with the active assistance and direction of the school physicians and the teachers; and 8) appeals to landlords throughout the county to improve living conditions.

024. Harris, Seale. "Tuberculosis in the Negro," Journal of the American Medical Association 41 (14) (October 3, 1903):834-838.

Observes that tuberculosis was a rare disease among the slaves in the southern states, yet after a quarter of a century it caused more deaths among emancipated blacks than all other infectious diseases. Attributes the situation to poor habits and sanitary conditions which are a result of blacks' indolence and improvidence. Points out studies which suggest that blacks have smaller lungs and less developed brains which are suggested as the reasons that blacks succumb to diseases such as tuberculosis. Recommends education, increasing the strength and vitality of the race, and isolation of those infected.

025. Hazen, H. H. "Personal Observations on Two Thousand Cases of Skin Disease in the Negro," Journal of the American Medical Association 62 (25) (June 20, 1914):1898.

A summary of a presentation to the American Dermatological Association, May, 1914, in Chicago. States that "The skin diseases more prevalent among negroes than white persons are dermatitis, papillaris capilliti, keloids, dry seborrhea, syphilis, tinea tonsurans, urticaria and vitilligo. Alopecia areata, cancer, eczema, erythema, furuncles, and boils, angiomas and nevi, Pediculus capitis and psoriasis are less prevalent among negroes than among white persons."

026. Hazen, H. H. "Syphilis in the American Negro," Journal of the American Medical Association 63 (6) (August 8, 1914):463-466.

Notes that the subject of syphilis in blacks is one that has not been thoroughly studied and, as a result, has led to many disputes and broad observations. In the past the tendency has been to publish personal opinions, often unaccompanied by evidence. Presents data from admissions to Freedmen's Hospital in Washington, D.C. from 1901 to 1912 and from personal experience. Discusses the various way that syphilis manifests itself and the difference between blacks and whites. Identifies two classes of the race, those who are trying to make something of themselves and the poor. It is the latter that is addressed in the paper. To reduce the problem of syphilis calls for study of the home problem, prevention of overcrowding, opportunities to live in decent dwellings and for changes in the delivery of medical care to individuals with syphilis.

027.   "Health Campaign Among Negroes," American Journal of Public Health 7 (Summer 1917):510.

In order to combat the unnecessarily high death rate among blacks, the New York City Department of Health, in cooperation with the National League on Urban Conditions among Blacks conducted an intensive educational campaign in that city for two weeks. Addressed was the black death rate was 24.4 for every 1,000 as compared to 13.7 per 1,000 for the rest of the population. Black babies born in the city have only half a chance of living through the first year than white babies.

028.   Hedrich, A. W.   "Cleaning Up the Negro Section," American Journal of Public Health 8 (Fall 1918):459.

In response to the very high death rate among the black population, the author, along with other members of the community, decided that educational work should be pushed, and a special colored visiting nurse was employed for work. Leaflets and other printed matter on health were distributed in black homes, lectures were given in black schools and churches, and house to house visits were made by the nurse instructing blacks in health and sanitary matters. Four years later, a marked decline in the local black death rate had occurred.

029.   Herrick, S. S.   "The Comparative Vital Movement of the White and Colored Races in the United States," Public Health Reports 7 (1881): 266-269.

The relative vital movement of different races in a mixed population was a matter of interest to the sanitarian as well as the ethnologist. It was found in this study that the mortality rate among "colored" people was higher among blacks than among whites. Pulmonary and other respiratory diseases were more detrimental to the black race. However, the black was less likely to contract cancerous diseases. As for diarrheal and puerperal diseases, whites had the upper hand. Attributes the better mortality rate to better medical attention and "superior" comforts of life that whites enjoy.

030.   Hess, Alfred F. and Unger, Lester J.   "Prophylactic Therapy for Rickets in a Negro Community," Journal of the American Medical Association 69 (19) (November 10, 1917):1583-1586.

A paper read before the Section on Prevention Medicine and Public Health at the American Medical Association meeting in June, 1917. Presents a study of black children who were subject to rickets to judge the effects of therapeutic doses of cod liver oil as a

prophylactic therapy. Fifty children between 4 months
and a year were the subjects of the study. Rickets were
prevented in four-fifths of the infants who receive the
oil for six months, and in one-half of those who
received it for four months. After the start of the
study, arrangements were made for the mothers to pick up
the oil rather than having it delivered. As a result,
word got around and the symptoms of rickets became
common knowledge and other mothers began to bring their
babies for consultation and cod liver oil. As a result,
a rickets clinic evolved. Dr. Haven Emerson of New
York, in commenting on the study, notes that what had
been thought of as a racial susceptibility may be merely
a result of an economic habit.

031. Hess, Alfred F. and Unger, Lester J. "The Diet of the
Negro Mother in New York City," Journal of the American
Medical Association 70 (13) (March 30, 1918):900-902.

A study of the diets of black women who had children
with rickets. The purpose was to determine whether the
food of the infants as well as the mother played a role
in the development of rickets. The diets of
seventy-five mothers were deficient in fresh fruits and
vegetables. Concludes that diet may well alter the
metabolism of the mother and her offspring.

032. Hindman, S. S. "Syphilis Among Insane Negroes,"
American Journal of Public Health 5 (3) (1915):213-224.

Reviews several studies to show the incidence of
syphilis among blacks, especially those admitted to
hospitals for the insane. Notes that syphilis in blacks
had received little attention until the last few years.
Argues that 95 percent of the black race will most
likely contract syphilis or some other venereal disease.
Reports findings of a study of black and white
admissions to the Georgia State Sanitarium. Finds the
syphilis rate in blacks to be 3 times that of the
whites. Concludes that syphilis as a cause of insanity
in blacks is rapidly becoming one of the most important
public health questions in the South.

033. Hummel, E. M. "The Rarity of Tabetic and Paretic
Conditions of the Negro: A Case of Tabes in a Full-Blood
Negress," Journal of the American Medical Association 56 (22)
(June 3, 1911):1645-1646.

Observes that it is a matter of belief among
neurologists that the so-called parasyphilitic
conditions--tabes and paresis--do not occur in the
full-blood African. Presents a case of tabes in a
full-blood black with the history and documentation of
the illnesses in the patient. Also discusses various
theories as to why full-blood blacks do not get the
disease. One theory has to do with the neurological and
neuromuscular development. The author believes that the
pressures and stresses of life lowers one's resistance

to the disease. Another theory is that the disease is prominent among blue or gray eyed blonds.

034. "Hygiene Among the Negro Population," <u>American Journal of Public Health</u> 5 (February 1915):81.

A brief discussion of the nature and work of the Negro Organization Society. This society is endeavoring to bring about better social and industrial conditions by instruction and cooperation along sanitary, hygienic, sociological and moral lines. Special attention is paid to matters of health, cleanliness and sanitary conditions. In these areas the organization is valuable to the white race as well as the black race since the positions of so many blacks in the servant class make improvement in matters of health a very important consideration.

035. "The Incidence of Disease Contrasted for White and Colored Troops," <u>Journal of the American Medical Association</u> 72 (20) (May 17, 1919):1468-1469.

A comment discussing research which compares white men and black men in the United States Army. Notes that the troops live under equally good sanitary conditions and are examined with equal diagnostic skill. A summary of the research is presented with differences between races being noted in a number of different diseases. Concludes that "in many respects the uninfected colored troops show themselves to be constitutionally better physiological machines than the white men."

036. Jones, Frank A. "Cardiac Lesions as Observed in the Negro, With Special Reference to Pericarditis," <u>Journal of the American Medical Association</u> 37 (24) (December 14, 1901):1581-1583.

Reviews a number of diseases based upon personal observations of 25,000 blacks over a five year period. Compares the research on cardiac lesions to personal observations, which are different. With reference to purulent pericarditis presents two cases as examples of the many that come under personal care, an eight year old black girl and a seventy-six year old black man. Provides a list of cardiac lesions in blacks in order of their frequency.

037. Jones, Frank A. "Cocaine Habit Among the Negroes," <u>Journal of the American Medical Association</u> 35 (3) (July 21, 1900):175.

A letter to the editor in response to an editorial in <u>The Journal</u> ("The Cocaine Habit," 34 (25) June 23, 1900, 1637). Reports on cocaine use in Memphis and notes that two-thirds of blacks addicted to cocaine use the "sniffing" method. Argues that the habit leads to acute mania and "The cocaine habit is one of the greatest evils to which the negro is addicted." "The cocaine sniffer is found among the lowest and most ignorant

class, both black and white. The evil is growing all
the time in Memphis." Reports a new ordinance in
Memphis which requires a certificate from a physician to
buy cocaine. The law also details what is included on
the certificate. Violation of the law for physicians
who write certificates for individuals for reasons other
than medical purposes is a fine of not less than $2.00
or more than $50.00.

038. Jones, Frank A. "Some Superstitions Among the Southern
Negroes," Journal of the American Medical Association 50 (15)
(April 11, 1908): 1207.

A letter to the editor detailing three superstitions
among southern blacks. 1) A live frog worn against the
throat for relief of a sore throat; 2) Bed bug tea (made
from live bed bugs) to "drive the de'ruption out"
(measles); 3) A full blown magnolia blossom inserted
into the vagina to treat leucorrhea.

039. Lee, Lawrence. "The Negro as a Problem in Public
Health Charity," American Journal of Public Health 5 (March
1915):194-203.

Identifies syphilis as the most important factor in the
high death rate of blacks. The living conditions of
blacks is seen as a major contributing factor. Fear of
ventiliation and over-crowding are reasons why
tuberculosis and respiratory diseases are so prevalent.
Notes that with education, blacks can become better
citizens, more useful members of the community and live
in better homes and more healthy surroundings.

040. Lofton, Lucien. "The Negro As A Surgical Subject."
New Orleans Medical and Surgical Journal 54 (February 1902):
530-533.

Discusses blacks as candidates for any surgical
technique and describes how blacks have been prone to
positive post-surgery results. Points out that
contaminated blood is the rule rather than the exception
among blacks which is due to the high rate of syphilis
and the negligence on the part of most blacks to have it
fully eradicated. Also observes that shock is not as
common in blacks as in whites because of the size of the
arteries and veins in blacks. Concludes that the black
diet, clothing and natural laws could be held ,
accountable if it were not for the fact that blacks eat,
sleep and work basically in the same manner and fashion
as whites. Notes that "Surgically everything is against
the Negro, physically he is operable, and without a
peer."

041. McDonald, Arthur. "Colored Children: A Psychophysical
Study," Journal of the American Medical Association 32 (21)
(May 27, 1899): 1140-1144.

Presents two original studies in which various measurements of colored children were obtained and compared to white children. The first study used an esthesiometer to measure the degree of ability to distinguish points on the skin by the sense of touch and a thermesthesiometer to distinguish difference in sensation of heat. The study used 91 black children and who were rated bright, average or dull by their teachers. Differences between bright and dull, boys and girls, whites and blacks were noted and reported. The second study of 5,457 black students used measurements made by teachers. Physical (height, sitting height, weight and circumference of the head) and mental (arithmetic, drawing, geography, history, language and english, music, penmanship, reading and spelling) measurements were obtained. The results were reported in tables. One finding reported was that the black children increased in brightness as age increased, whereas white children decreased in brightness as age increased. Concludes that the cause of this difference in black children was racial.

042. Mckie, Thomas J. "A Brief History of Insanity and Tuberculosis in the Southern Negro," Journal of the American Medical Association 28 (12) (March 20, 1897):537-538.

A brief personal historical account of the development of tuberculosis and insanity in a small area going back to 1848. Notes the first case of the diseases and the spread and presents personal observations as to the etiology and the reasons for the sudden and unaccountable increase of tuberculosis in blacks. Speculated on life style, but notes that the well-to-do families supplied the greater number of insane and tuberculosis subjects. Concludes that insanity and tuberculosis are allied diseases, and that "both...in the Southern Negro are the outcome of an overtaxed and overworked nervous organization unfitted by nature and otherwise to bear the burden imposed by newly created necessities or environment; that insanity and tuberculosis are primarily and essentially neuroses."

043. McVey, Bruce "Negro Practice," New Orleans Medical and Surgical Journal 20 (November 1882): 328-332.

Discusses differences between black patients and white patients. Notes that blacks are stoutier and heartier than whites and that habit and environment can affect the outcome of drug therapy. Also discusses consumption and the lack of this disease in blacks that lived in the country versus the presence of the disease in those blacks that lived in small towns. Concludes by discussing the prevalence of venereal disease in blacks and the problems associated with treatment.

044. Meyers, Sarah B. "The Negro Problem as it Appears to a Public Health Nurse," The American Journal of Nursing 19 (1918):278-281.

Begins with the observation "No greater task confronts the south to-day (sic) than that of converting the southern negro into a being who recognizes the laws of health and sanitation..." Explains how white homes are be infected with diseases because of the total lack of healthy conditions and practices among blacks who serve in the homes of whites. For this reason argues that whites should take an interest in improving blacks' cleanliness, mode of living and knowledge and disease prevention. Presents self experiences on visiting the 'negro quarters' in Fulton, Kentucky and the successes in improving their living conditions. Describes the personal relationships developed with several blacks and involvement in establishing a Red Cross Chapter among blacks and the involvement of blacks in chapter.

045. Miller, Kelly. "The Historic Background of the Negro Physician," Journal of Negro History 1 (2) (1916): 99-109.

Discusses the ways in which race complicates "every feature of the social equation." Devotes some attention to the control of disease through roots, herbs, charms and conjurations practiced in Africa and transported to America, referring to a black medicine man named Cesar whose cure for poison is footnoted on one half of the page. Circumstances concerning Cesar's freedom are also mentioned. Also, discusses the role of slaves in a doctor-like capacity includes a runaway slave named Simon who was advertised as "pretending to be a great doctor among his people" as well as a fugitive slave about whom Charleston, South Carolina's City Gazette and Daily Advertiser said "He passes for a Doctor among people of his color...." Slaves who were barbers, took on the trade of a physician. Joseph Ferguson, knowledgable as a lecher, cupper, and barber led to his study of medicine around 1861. He practiced in Michigan after his graduation. Notes the rise of the first formally trained black physicians who practiced in the United States including James Denham, James McCune Smith and others and the important role of several organizations in bringing blacks into the medical profession.

046. Murrell, Thomas W. "Syphilis and the American Negro," Journal of the American Medical Association 54 (11) (March 12, 1910):846-849.

Offers insight into the conditions confronting blacks as they relates to syphilis through a sociological presentation with the changes that have occurred as a result of freedom and the impact it had on the spread of the disease. Discusses data showing the increasing rate of infection and death. Predicts syphilis will continue to spread and in fifty years it will be difficult to find an unsyphilic black. Also discusses the physical symptoms of the disease as they relate to blacks. Recommends not using treatment causing pain as it is unlikely that blacks will show up for a second treatment. Argues that teaching blacks the hygiene of the disease is hopeless and laws must be made that relate to blacks and only blacks, similar to laws made for the Indian.

047.   "The National Negro Antituberculosis League," Journal of the American Medical Association 52 (12) (March 20, 1909):969.

An editorial that announces a new organization sponsored by the Public Health and Marine-Hospital Service of the U.S. recently inaugurated in Savannah, Georgia. Reviews the history of tuberculosis in the black race and factors which led to its increase. Describes the organization as one "which shall bring them together on the basis of instruction in sanitation and right-living and will surely aid in checking the advancing scourge of tuberculosis among them."

048.   "The Negro and Public Health," American Journal of Public Health 4 (May 1914):624-625.

In response to the suggestion that blacks may stand in another relation to public health other than merely as a menace to society is indicated in an effort conducted by a number of prominent black leaders in Virginia. Over 130,000 heads of black families engaged in a cleanup of living areas of a number of black communities. The areas cleaned up represented some of the worst living conditions where disease was rampant. The trash drive received unusual cooperation from the State Board of Health, white newspapers, and other agencies. The effort was aimed at not only benefitting blacks, but whites as well.

049.   "The Negro As Asset and Liability." New Orleans Medical and Surgical Journal 67 (October 1914): 384-385.

Addresses some issues regarding health conditions among blacks that were raised at a conference of physicians. Argues that it is no longer necessary for health boards to be comprised entirely of white physicians because of black intermingling with whites. Discusses education, disease (Syphilis, etc.) and morality and how each is related to black health care. Concludes by noting that unless restructuring of the black economic existence occurs, both races are destined for destruction.

050.   "The Negro Menace to the Public Health," American Journal of Public Health 6 (Summer 1916):607.

Referencing an article that appeared in the Southern Medical Journal, reports that Dr. Graves points out four lines along which the most progress can probably be made in the improvement of the blacks' condition: the enactment of proper housing laws, education for both races, instituting certain legal and social restrictions, and providing public clinics in all municipalities large enough to bear the expense for medical, surgical and dental service to the poor and ignorant.

051.   Powell, Theophilus O.   "The Increase of Insanity and Tuberculosis in the Southern Negro Since 1860, and Its Alliance, and Some of the Supposed Causes," Journal of the American Medical Association 27 (December 5, 1896):1185-1188.

The author discusses the numbers of insane blacks in Georgia taken from the censuses of 1860, 1870, 1880, and 1890 and links insanity with tuberculosis. Describes the causes for the rapid increase of these two 'diseases' and others among Southern blacks. Notes the excellent health conditions on plantations prior to emancipation due to owners' interest in keeping a healthy working force. Argues that after 1865, the deterioration in sanitation, the lack of a systematic and regular life, the lack of restraint from excesses (including alcoholism), the syphilis carry over from slavery and the fact that blacks worked in Southern institutions where whites with tuberculosis resided are the primary causes of the increases in insanity and tuberculosis among blacks.

052.   Reyburn, R.   "Types of Disease Among the Freed People (mixed Negro race) of the United States," Medical News (1893):623-627.

The years immediately following the Civil War produced a new interest in general black related social issues and among these were health issues. A study based on the consolidated reports of over 430,466 cases of sick and wounded free people of mixed African descent and compared with 22,053 similar cases involving white refugees who were under treatment between the end of the war in 1865 until the end of June 1872 from the Federal Bureau of Refugees, Freedmen and Abandoned Lands.

053.   Sheppegrell, W.   "The Comparative Pathology of the Negro," Proceedings of the Orleans Parish Medical Society (1896):589-593.

A study of 11,855 black patients with ear, nose and throat ailments reported to the Orleans Parish Medical Society.

054.   Springarn, Arthur B.   "The War and Venereal Disease Among Negroes," Social Hygiene 4 (2) (April 1918): 333-346.

Concerned with the medical activities aimed at the prevention and treatment of venereal disease among black troops in the camps and with the infection in the civil communities accessible to the military forces. Contends the selective drafts does not allow Americans to ignore the health problem of the black, since nearly 10 percent of the military are selected from black ranks. Venereal disease is the greatest single factor in the non-effective rate of the army, and its incidence is greater among black troops than among white. The problem must be addressed from the viewpoint of the potential as well as the actual soldier. Inevitably, every influence that makes for morality within the power of the white to withhold from the black has been withheld. The black girl has less education, less legal protection, lives under less sanitary conditions, have less recreational opportunities, a lower economic status, is the prey of men of both races, and is no better off than her mother. For every safeguard that is placed about the white girl, there is a corresponding obstacle thrown in the black girl's path. This and more add up to a higher venereal rate among blacks. Concludes that there should be equal and adequate medical treatment for the black soldier, a place for him to go for decent recreation, both inside and outside camp. The black community should be organized and a special education campaign on social hygiene should be made for black soldiers and civilians. Also, adequate and equal law enforcement should be obtained for blacks and whites and equal clinical and hospital facilities and rehabilitation and detention of black girls should be established immediately.

055. Stone, I. S. "The Rarity of Ovarian Cysts in Negresses," Journal of the American Medical Association 31 (26) (December 24, 1898):1530.

A summary of a paper presented at the eleventh annual meeting of the Southern Surgical and Gynecological Association in 1898. After several years of treating gynecological diseases, the author notes extreme rarity of ovarian neoplasms, especially of the multilocular variety. Presents survey findings from members of the association and several prominent surgical hospitals and finds support for this theory, except one hospital in New Orleans which found cysts more frequently in blacks than in whites. Concludes that ovarian cysts are exceedingly rare in black women.

056. Talbot, Eugene S. "Etiology of Face, Nose and Jaw Deformities," Journal of the American Medical Association 52 (13) (March 27, 1909):1020-1021.

A systematic investigation was started in 1874 to ascertain the character and determine the classification of deformities of the head, face, jaws and teeth. Although the study was extensive, one area of investigation dealt with facial evolution. Argues that when the forehead, face and jaws are on the perpendicular line this is indicative of man's evolution. Reports a study of an examination of blacks of the lower type in Mississippi which indicated that 97.5 percent had jaws that extended beyond the perpendicular line, while an examination of 10,000 people on the streets of London revealed only 4.13 percent of the cases had jaws that extended beyond the line. Out of 1,000 blacks in Boston, only 45.4 percent had jaws that extended beyond the line, and in Chicago, out of 2,000 cases, only 6 had dolichocephalic heads.

Uses these figures to suggest that evolution had occurred in the black race in the last 250 years since coming to the United States.

057. Taylor, J. Madison. "The Negro and His Health Problems." Medical Records (September 1912): 513-515.

The black health problem is one of characteristical heredity. Although it does involve such issues as economics, improper hygiene, and lack of education, these factors should not be considered exclusively. The black problem is one of displacement from his natural environment. Accustomed to tropical climates, the black has been situated in an environment that lacks adequate sunshine, ventilation and space necessary to fit his character. The original blacks brought over from Africa as slaves had a much higher tolerance for disease than their lineage due to hybrids. After coming in contact with whites, the black experienced a dilution of his character resulting from the sexual union of the different races. However, there are remedies to the black health problems. First, the black must be educated as to the proper health laws. He must be taught self respect and obedience. Many blacks dwell in homes with poor ventilation. In his native land he was accustomed to wide open spaces. The black in the South is therefore less susceptable to disease than his counterpart from the Northern cities. His situation is less drastically changed than his counterpart. He may dwell in solitude of others. However, blacks in Northern cities dwell in crowded facilities with improper sanitation. Black role models must be established to present them with proper methods of sanitation and hygiene. They must be placed strategically so as to be of the best use. They must remove the educational limitations prohibiting adequate health status.

058. Terry, C. E. "The Negro: His Relation to Public Health in the South." American Journal of Public Health 3 (1913): 300-10.

The author is a medical doctor from Jacksonville, Florida. Observes that black health should be improved, if for no other reason, to prevent the spread of communicable diseases to whites. Provides data from Jacksonville that indicate that the rate of black mortality is higher than that of whites. Blacks are particularly hard hit by malaria, whooping cough, influenze, tuberculosis of the lungs, venereal diseases, pneumonia, diarrhea, and congenital debility. A large degree of the high mortality rates can be attributed to ignorance of black midwives, lack of sanitary education in the black community, and a distrust of white doctors in the black community. Argues that charity extended to the blacks is not enough. Municipal health departments must see to mosquito extermination and, when necessary, must extend some help in providing privies and digging wells.

059. Thornton, G. B. "The Negro Mortality in Memphis,"
Public Health: Reports and Papers of the American Public
Health Association 8 (1882): 177-186.

Examines the data of the 1880 census to demonstrate the
equal population figures for blacks and whites in
Memphis, and then goes beyond those figures to discuss
why in 1882 blacks suffer a disproportionately high
mortality rate that is fifty percent higher than for
Memphis whites. Notes that blacks seldom suffer from
chorea and epilepsy, and suffer from acute insanity less
often than do whites. Thornton notes that blacks do
possess a "mental obliquity" that is a form of monomania
and which manifests itself in superstitious beliefs that
can be injurious to his health. Ultimately, poor black
mortality is due to ignorant midwives, improper labor
management, and a licentious mode of life.

060. Trask, John W. "The Significance of the Mortality
Rates of the Colored Population of the United States,"
American Journal of Public Health 6 (January 1916):254-259.

Those interested in the public health of blacks should
be concerned with the difference between the white and
black death rates. The reasons for the differences,
whether the cause is an essential one inherent in one
element of the population and not in the other, whether
the factors which produce the difference in the death
rates can be removed, and the colored death rate lowered
are discussed.

061. Walton, J. T. "The Comparative Mortality of the White
and Colored Races in the South," Charlotte Medical Journal 10
(1897): 291-294.

Since emancipation the health status of blacks has
declined drastically. Data reveal that the black
mortality rate is twice that of Whites. Blacks seem to
have become susceptible to diseases their bodies were
once capable of warding off. One such disease is
Consumption. Southern physicians have noted that in pre
Ante-bellum days, Consumption in blacks was a rarity and
nearly never seen. As a slave, the black man seemed
more than sturdy and a physical specimen to behold.
However, his emancipation marks not only his freedom but
his decline. Data from a number of Southern cities
reveal that between 1854-1865 the death rate was much
larger in whites than blacks. However, since his
freedom, the table has turned. Data also reveal that
the majority of blacks who die from Consumption are of
lighter skin. The black disease problem can be
attributed to general ignorance, lack of proper food and
clothing, improper ventilated dwellings, inadequate
medical attention and insanitary living surroundings.

062. Wilson, Jr., Robert. "Some Medical Aspects of the
Negro." Southern Medical Association (1915): 3-6.

Remarks given by the author as chairman of the Section
on Medicine of the Southern Medical Association's eighth
annual meeting held in Richmond, Virginia. The remarks
briefly point out the importance of blacks from the
medical viewpoint and urges doctors to become
knowledgeable of blacks' medical characteristics which
indicate possibly profitable lines of study. Referring
to some of the research, he acknowledges the dearth of
accurate knowledge and states that some of the
conceptions are only unproved assumptions. It is
clearly the duty of doctors to determine if commonly
accepted beliefs are true and to determine their impact
on the community. Blacks have brought with them
diseases affecting public health. Some of these include
leprosy, hemoglobinusic fever, filareasis, uncinariasis,
and yellow fever. Blacks have become a great carrier of
tuberculosis. Several writers indicate that blacks are
more susceptible to malaria than whites and research is
being done on the Negro as a carrier of filarial
infection. Medically considered, blacks' extremely high
mortality from combined cardio-vascular-renal diseases
is one of the most striking features. In order to study
blacks, urges separation of blacks and mulattoes as well
as careful, comprehensive clinical observations followed
by laboratory and post-mortem investigation.

2

THE LITERATURE FROM
1920 TO 1950

063. "A Ghetto Destroyed." Time 58 (August 23, 1954): 58.

Calls attention to encouraging news on the medical front. At the convention of the National Medical Association, a professional organization of U.S. black physicians, it was noted that the 'walls' of discrimination were falling. In 1947 black medical graduates could hope to interne in only a few hospitals, most of them segregated. The numbers were far from desirable, but the so called 'ghetto plan' for providing health care for blacks was being destroyed.

064. "A National Organization for the Health of Negro Students," Journal of Social Hygiene 21 (7-8-9) (October, November, December 1935):375.

In October of 1934, black colleges formed an organization known as the National Negro Student Health Association, which worked closely with the American Social Health Association. Officers of the new National Negro Student Health Association were: Dr. Paul B. Cornely, Howard University and Franklin O. Nichols. The purpose of the new organization was to raise the standards of student health service in black colleges; to develop further progress in health matters in black institutions; and to afford better cooperation to established health agencies desiring to reach these colleges. Several committees of the Association dealt with syphilis, tuberculosis, health education, sight conversation, and standards of student health services. The Association also conducted a thorough tuberculosis case-finding program in black colleges, with the aid and cooperation of black school physicians.

065. "A Study of the Attitude of a Group of Male Negroes Toward Venereal Disease," Venereal Disease Information 5 (4) (April 1924): 175-176.

A survey to determine the attitudes of a group of black males toward venereal disease and to measure the knowledge of the group concerning venereal disease. The results of this survey are of particular interest to those who carry out a program of venereal disease control. The survey found a high incidence of venereal

disease among the blacks questioned. Fifty-four percent
of those responding indicated an experience with
gonorrhea while eight percent had an experience with
syphilis. The average incidence of gonorrhea among the
respondents was 1.7 times. The survey also indicated
ignorance of important information concerning the
transmittal of gonorrhea. Many of the men in the survey
did not believe that the male can transmit gonorrhea to
the female. A third of those diseased reported having
sexual intercourse before the infection cleared up.
Concludes by stressing that the gonorrhea infection rate
for black professionals is nearly half that of black
nonprofessionals.

066. Abbott, Grace. "Methods by Which Children's Health May
be Improved," Opportunity 2 (13) (January 1924): 10-11.

In an address before the National Urban League
Conference in Kansas City, Missouri on October 18, 1923,
the author stresses the importance of the health of the
black child. Observes that in 1921 the infant mortality
rate for blacks in the birth registration area of the
United States was 108 as compared to 72 for whites. In
a series of studies of infant mortality made by the
Children's Bureau, it was found that poverty was the
black child's greatest enemy. Contends that the
handicap of poverty can be overcome if there is made
available for the mother information as to: (1) what
constitutes good care for herself before and during
childbirth and (2) what constitutes good care for the
baby. Discusses comparisons between the infant
mortality rates of whites and blacks from 1915 - 1921 in
both urban and rural areas and also briefly discusses
the causes and effects of rickets to children and the
preventive work necessary to resist them. Notes reports
showing that black mothers are more easily persuaded to
adopt good methods of child care than white mothers of
the same educational and economic levels.

067. Abbott, Grace. "A Message to Colored Mothers," Crisis
39 (10) (October 1932):311-312, 332.

Emphasizes that despite the "handicaps" black mothers
must endure to insure their children are healthy, they
have made great progress. By 1932 the general trend of
the infant death rate in America had declined. This
downward trend may be credited "to mothers who have
given more scientific care to their children and
utilized more intelligently the knowledge and the skill
which the doctor has to offer." Concludes that medical
advances and parental involvement, particularly that of
the mother, will greatly improve the health of children.

068. Adams, Numa P. G. "Sources of Supply of Negro Health
Personnel: Physicians," Journal of Negro Education 6
(1937):468-76.

Discusses the decline in the number of black medical
students from 510 in 1927 to 377 in 1935 and identifies

reasons for the decline. Stresses five needs that are
necessary before blacks can graduate from medical
schools in sufficient numbers. First, undergraduate
training facilities must be improved and postgraduate
education needs to be established at Howard and Meharry
medical schools. Second, medical schools in the North
must continue accepting qualified black students.
Third, scholarships and financial aid for black medical
students are necessary. Fourth, facilities for black
interns and residents must be improved. Finally, short
and intensive postgraduate courses for black doctors are
required in areas of the country in which specific
expertise is needed. The author was Dean of the School
of Medicine at Howard University.

069. Adams, Walter A. "The Negro Patient in Psychiatric
Treatment," American Journal of Orthopsychiatry 20 (2) (April
1950):305-310.

Emphasizes the importance of white psychiatrists
assuming the responsibility and acquiring the techniques
and skills necessary in order to handle mental illness
among blacks. Argues that therapists "who accept Negro
patients must examine with considerable care their
attitudes and feelings toward race, and they should also
possess a knowledge of the structure and cultural
background of the Negro social groups." Unlike white
patients, black patients may become offended by semantic
errors made by the therapist. Argues that the therapist
"should see himself as potentially threatening to the
patient at many levels, not only because of his
(patient's) subordinate position with reference to class
but also because dynamically he represents a parental
figure in the transference situation, more wholesomely
identified symbolically as a mature father, a mature
mother or older sibling." In other words,
"preconditioned fear and distrust of the original father
may be displaced through transference on to dislike of
the racial stranger." Concludes "in order to reach his
Negro patient's more basic personality problems, the
white therapist must penetrate those defenses which may
be expressed in racial conflict." Recognizes the need
for an improved social system based on justice and
fairness to minorities by making therapist realize the
need to draw the mentally sick black patient away from
his rationalizations.

070. Aery, William Anthony. "Conserving Negro Lives,"
Southern Workman (September 1936): 282-284.

The article discusses midwifery and practical nursing
and is based on a report of the Doctors' Helpers
Institute, which was held at the Hampton Institute. The
Institute taught women how to give nursing services in
rural communities and doctors gave talks to the women
attending, especially on pre-natal and post-natal care.
Demonstrations then followed on bed-making techniques,
preparing baths for babies, procedures to prepare for a
delivery, giving enemas, and etc. Women from ten

Virginia counties participated in this program. The
Institute seeks to provide training to doctors' helpers
and midwives to reduce deaths among black mothers and
their infants.

071. Alexander, Virginia and Simpson, George E.   "Negro
Hospitalization," Opportunity 15 (8) (August 1937): 231-232.

During the third Institute of Race Relations Conference
held at Swarthmore College in July of 1935, under the
auspices of the American Friends Service Committee, a
study of the health problems of North Philadelphia
blacks was made. A summary of the findings is presented
which shows concretely the discriminatory practices
taking place with regard to black hospitalization in
North Philadelphia. Some of the findings include the
following: (1) blacks are not admitted to some wards in
some hospitals; (2) black doctors frequently encounter
hostile attitudes from white physicians; and (3) there
is no opportunity in all Philadelphia for a black
physician to get experience or training in contagious
diseases or in neuropsychiatry. Makes recommendations
which could lead to improvement in this city as well as
others especially in the North.

072. "An All-Community Problem," Journal of Social Hygiene
10 (7) (October 1924): 426.

Praises the greater community appreciation of the mutual
dependence of different races on each other for better
health. There is an expanding realization of the fact
that diseases do not draw color lines. A disease must
be eliminated regardless of the race of the victim.
Still, there is much to be done in the community to
further reduce the morbidity and mortality rates among
blacks. Tuberculosis, venereal diseases and infantile
disorders are major killers of blacks. These conditions
will spread to the North as blacks steadily migrate
there and will have detrimental affects on the northern
industrial communities. Northern sections of the
country should give increased study to the situation in
order for the community to understand the problem of
blacks relative to disease so as to advise ways and
means for existing agencies to promote the public health
and social welfare of the community. Previous studies
indicate that the development and use of black personnel
to work in those social organizations aimed at educating
black communities to the facts concerning venereal
disease will be advantageous for the controlled handling
of the condition.

073. Allen, E. H. "Extending Health Horizons Among
Negroes," Opportunity 24 (June 1946):28-9.

During World War II, a million black youths were given
health analysis in the military. These men have been
better treated and are more conscious in regard to
tuberculosis, venereal diseases, dentistry, and surgical
care. These developments will be of great value to

young men with years of life ahead of them. The war has
aided the training of many black physicians, nurses,
dentists, and medical technicians.

074. Allen, Floyd P. "Physical Impairment Among One
Thousand Negro Workers," American Journal of Public Health 22
(June 1932):579-86.

A study of 1,000 black factory workers over age twenty
in Cincinnati supported by the Public Health Federation
and the Anti-Tuberculosis League of Cincinnati. Only
one of the thousand men examined was found to be free of
physical defects. Only eight men knew of their defects
prior to the examination. Over five hundred men had
significant cardiovascular abnormalities. Over two
hundred had hypertension. Among men under forty years
old, the greater the amount of overweight, the higher
the incidence of cardiovascular abnormalities found.
The outstanding communicable disease among Cincinnati
blacks was tuberculosis. The average age where
tuberculosis was either found or suspected was
thirty-seven years.

075. Altschul, Alexander and Nathan, Arthur. "Diabetes
Mellitus in Harlem Hospital Outpatient Department in New
York: A Comparison of Certain Etiologic Factors in Negro and
White Patients," Journal of the American Medical Association
119 (3) (May 16, 1942):248-252.

Discusses the disease diabetes mellitus in the black
community. Presents data indicating the higher
incidence of diabetes in the black female than any other
group and observes that the onset is earlier in the
black female than any other group.

076. "American College of Surgeons Admits Negro Candidates,"
Opportunity 25 (January 1949):29.

Describes how the American College of Surgeons was
charged with restricting its black membership in 1945.
To correct this practice, eight black candidates were
sent notices for initiation ceremonies in 1946. During
1945, Dr. George Thorne, a staff member of the Syndenham
Hospital, wrote for an application to the American
College of Surgeons Clinical Congress. He was informed
that fellowship in the College was not being conferred
on members of the black race at that time. Previously,
Dr. Louis T. Wright was the only black member, having
been inducted in 1934.

077. "American Medical Association Elects First Negro to
House of Delegates," National Negro Health News 18 (1)
(1950): 27.

Elections of a black physician to the American Medical
Association's House of Delegates was announced at the
annual meeting of the National Medical Association, a
black organization, in Detroit. The New York State
Medical Society had named Dr. Peter Marshall Murray,

Director of the Department of Gynecology at Harlem
Hospital, as one of its delegates to the national body,
and announced that Dr. Murray will be seated at the
annual meeting of the American Medical Association in
San Francisco next June. He is the first black
physician to become a member of the American Medical
Association policy-making group.

078.   "The American Red Cross and Negro Health." National
Negro Health News 15 (1) (January-March, 1947): 1-4.

Reports the increase in voluntary involvment of blacks
(primarily women) in health-care programs of The
American Red Cross. The stimulus for the survey of
black involvement in The American Red Cross programs
came from the recent example of the Volunteer Nurse's
Aid Corp at Mercy Hospital in St. Petersburg, Florida.
In order to show their willingness to get involved and
in order to improve health care for the patients at
Mercy Hospital (primarily a hospital for blacks) women
of the community underwent training programs and
voluntarily assisted in health care at the hospital.
The report includes lists of organizations and
activities in both civilian and veteran health
institutions in five other states as well. Areas in
which the increasing activity of blacks in health aid is
being felt include hospitals, clinics, schools, first
aid and safety training programs, nutrition schools, and
home nursing courses. All these programs were conducted
under the auspices of The Red Cross.

079. "An Experiment in Venereal Disease Education in Negro
Schools," The Journal of Venereal Disease Information 26 (11)
(November 1945): 245.

Discusses an experimental venereal disease information
program in seven Southern black schools in Georgia and
North Carolina. The information programs consists of
different combinations of posters, pamphlets and teacher
instruction. Finds that simple inexpensive methods of
information dissemination were effective and resulted in
a marked increase in the extent and accuracy of
knowledge among black students concerning venereal
disease. The gain among these test students ranged from
twenty to three-hundred percent. The net gain in
information per pupil ranged from 6.2 to 10.8 percent.

080.   Anderson, Peyton F.   "The Negro Tuberculosis Patient
and Surgical Treatment," National Negro Health News 3 (2)
(1935): 16-17.

With the advent of active surgical measures for the
treatment of tuberculosis, interest in this disease took
a sudden hopeful spurt forward in all of the more
enlightened countries of the world. This interest aided
all divisions of internal medicine, for with it came
better diagnoses. Whites and blacks agree that the
health of the blacks is largely the responsibility of
the black medical profession. That profession is

expected to reduce a disastrous death rate from
tuberculosis. But it cannot do this until its members
are given the opportunity not only of learning about
modern methods but also of carrying them out.

081. Anderson, Peyton F. and Peterson, Jerome S. "Warring
Against Tuberculosis in Harlem," Crisis 49 (11) (November
1942):356-359, 366.

Outlines the important work accomplished in the war
against the tuberculosis in the world's largest black
community, Harlem. By 1942 the Harlem Tuberculosis and
Health Committee, a public health project, had been in
service for twenty years. The Committee was organized
to improve health conditions of people living in Harlem.
Black nurses and physicians were trained to work in the
clinic. Dr. Henry Minton of Philadelphia was a black
physician actively involved in the war against
tuberculosis. The Committee's first step in combatting
tuberculosis in Harlem was to create an awareness of
leading disease problems in the community. Tuberculosis
received the most attention, since this disease ranked
high in Harlem as a cause of sickness or death. In
addition to combatting tuberculosis the Committee in
1924 set up a model dental clinic "as an educational
factor and as a demonstration of what would be done to
meet the need of dental hygiene for children and
prenatal mothers whose incomes do not permit private
care." The work of the Committee in combatting
tuberculosis in Harlem did improve the health of blacks.

082. "Announcement of 1947 National Negro Health Week,"
National Negro Health News 14 (3) (1946): 4.

The National Negro Health Week will be commemorated
between March 30 and April 6, 1947. Its special
objective will be "Community-Wide Cooperation for Better
Health and Sanitation." In general, the nation was
becoming more health conscious. The emphasis was now
upon effective health education and the provision of
adequate health facilities and health services. The
1947 Health Week publications - Bulletin, poster and
school leaflet - will be ready for distribution in the
early part of next year. The October - December, 1946
issue of the National Negro Health News, which will be
released in February, 1947, will carry suggestions for
community organization and activities. It will also
contain special articles on pertinent phases of the 1947
Health Week objective.

083. Austin, B. F. "Negro Health Problems," Health
Instruction 1943 Yearbook (1943):13-14.

Discusses the health problems of blacks in rural
Alabama. In all of the diseases common to people in
this area, blacks have consistently higher incidence of
occurrence than whites: whooping cough death rate is 2½
times as high; tuberculosis death rate is 3 times as
high; malaria death rate is twice as high; syphilis

death rate is 7 times as high; and brain hemorrhages are 53 percent more frequent among blacks.

084. Baker, Benjamin M. "Certain Aspects of Syphilitic Cardiac Disease," Venereal Disease Information 12 (September 20, 1931): 471.

The history of the knowledge of syphilitic cardiac disease is examined in this article. Additionally, the admissions to Johns Hopkins Hospital from January 1, 1918 to February 20, 1930 were also examined. As discovered by the author, among the 20,893 patients admitted to Johns Hopkins Hospitals, 17,126 were white and 3,761 were black. Among the 2,196 cases of syphilis, 488 were cases of cardiac syphilis (aorta). Of the 969 syphilitic blacks, 317 had syphilis of the aorta. Of the 1,227 syphilitic whites, 171 had aorta syphilis. It was concluded that the mortality rate was twice as high for syphilitic heart disease than from other heart diseases. This leads the author to conclude that many more Negroes would die from syphilis than whites.

085. Bakwin, Harry. "The Negro Infant," Human Biology 4 (February 1932): 1-33.

It was the purpose of this paper to assemble data on the differences between black and white infants in good health and with disease, and to determine to what extent these differences were dependent upon race. Measles was found to be as often a cause of death among Negroes as among white infants. In later life, measles were less common in blacks. Scarlet fever was found to be less common among blacks than among white infants. Whooping cough was more than twice as common a cause of death in blacks than in white infants. Diphtheria was a more common cause of death among black infants that among white infants. Syphilis was much more prevalent in blacks that in white infants. There were no reports indicating racial differences in the disease manifestations such as seen in the adult. Influenza, like other respiratory infections, was more fatal in blacks than in white infants. According to the author, the mortality rate for the black infant was much higher than for the white infant. The infant death rate from pneumonia (all forms) was almost twice as high in blacks as in whites. The death rate for birth injuries was considerably lower in blacks than in white infants. Research finds that the death rate and disease has a definite race link.

086. Bakwin, H. and Bakwin, Ruth Morris. "The Dosage of Ultraviolet Radiation in Infants with Tetany," Journal of the American Medical Association 95 (6) (August 9, 1930): 396-399.

A study of the effects of different dosages of ultraviolet radiation in the treatment of infants with tetany. A total of 28 children were studied, 14 white and 14 colored (9 blacks, 4 Puerto Ricans, and 1

Filipino) using 3 dosages, low, optimal and high.
Within the optimal and high ranges, there was no
difference in response between the 3 groups. Within the
low dosage range, the white infants responded at a more
rapid rate than the black children. Concludes that a
greater minimal dose is necessary for the cure of tetany
in black children than is necessary in white children.

087. Bakwin, H. and Patrick, T. W. "The Weight of Negro
Infants," Journal of Pediatrics 24 (1944): 405-407.

A study conducted on 114 black infants seen in private
practice and supervised from early life by one of the
authors. Based on findings and comparisons with
accepted observations of white infants. Concludes that
there are no significant differences between the weight
gain of white and black infants when fed the same stable
complex diet.

088. Bartholomew, R. A. "Syphilis as a Complication of
Pregnancy in the Negro," Journal of the American Medical
Association 83 (3) (July 19, 1924):172-174.

Notes that analyses of the deaths of stillborn or full
term babies (up to the first two weeks of life) show
that syphilis is the cause of death in a third of the
cases and that there is an usually high incidence of
syphilis among black obstetric patients. Using
admissions during 1922 and 1923 of black obstetric
patients, compares 100 syphilitic and 100 nonsyphilitic
patients and finds three times as many abortions and
premature labors, and seventeen times as many
stillbirths in the syphilitic as in the nonsyphilitic.
Also compares 100 untreated syphilitic patients with 100
treated syphilitic patients (treatment from an average
of 7.4 months on to the end of pregnancy) and finds that
premature births are twice as frequent, stillbirths
three times as frequent, abortions seven times as
frequent, and infant deaths nine times as frequent in
the untreated versus the treated patients. Recommends
that clinics make use of all means of diagnosis in order
to arrive at a true estimate of the importance of
syphilis as a factor in fetal mortality.

089. Beck, Samuel J. "The Rorschach Test in a Case of
Character Neurosis," American Journal of Orthopsychiatry 14
(2) (April 1944):230-236.

Presents a case history and Rorschach analysis of an
American black man to show the clear relationship
between clinical material and test responses. The
purpose of the study is to demonstrate that the test
results are valid for this American because he is a
product of American culture and this factor overrides
the importance of race. "The Rorschach test shows here
that, given constancy of culture, the fact of race is of
less importance in the final product, and therefore the
adult personality structure in this American Negro is a
mold of his environment." The author's findings rebut

the argument that a different Rorschach pattern should
be looked for in a black. The black patient who has
been "brought up in North American culture, is subjected
to the cultural climate... with regard to ambition,
education, the 'duty to get rich,' and our other
vagaries."

090. Beckham, Albert Sidney. "Applied Eugenics," Crisis 28
(4) (August 1924):177-178.

Advocates eugenics, the science of improving the race
through better heredity. Argues that "selective mating"
will improve the mental, moral, and physical development
of the race and that eugenics would increase the mental
level of blacks. Argues that eugenics could aid "the
greatest problems of the twentieth century, that of the
Negro" and while eugenics may not solve racial ills, "it
is a pathway that leads to the solving of a number of
racial problems with which we have to contend."
Concludes that "persons of like undesirable traits
should not mate" and "Persons of the best blood as
evident by mental, moral, and physical life should mate
if possible." For example, "when both parents lack the
capacity of developing properly the cortical cells, all
the children will be wanting in that respect; such
individuals should not marry.

091. Bender, L. "Behavior Problems in Negro Children,"
Psychiatry 2 (2) (May 1939): 213-228.

It has been claimed that differences between whites and
blacks in mental and nervous disease exist due to actual
racial differences or to the primitivity of blacks.
More careful studies have tended to disprove such
differences in most cases. The differences have often
been accounted for on the basis of social and economical
conditions and of congenital anatomical variations in
size and development tendencies. There does seem to be
some evidence of a difference in the mesoderm which
leads to a different reactivity of the vascular-system
of blacks and may cause some special deviations in
organic brain condition related to hypertension and
perhaps syphilis. Otherwise there appears to be some
evidence for a greater range of deviation or a greater
coefficient of variability in certain structures and
function, such as the brain weight or intelligence
level. The number of black children brought for
observation to the Psychiatric Division of Bellevue
exceeds the expectancy when compared with the white
children. Mental deficiency does not account for this.
Neither does syphilis. Poor physical conditions are
traced to poor economical and social background which
tend to lower the child's psychobiological capacities
and add to the other factors that make the black child
feel inferior.

092. Bender, L. and Yarrell, Z. "Psychosis Among Followers
of Father Divine," The Journal of Nervous and Mental Diseases
87 (April 1938):418-419.

A study of the effects on the followers of the
controversial black charismatic religious leader of the
1920's with intent of establishing the level of mental
incompetence.

093.   Benjamin, Edward A. and Robertson, Thomas E.   "Some
Socioeconomic Aspects of Venereal Disease Among Negroes,"
National Negro Health News 16 (April-June 1948): 11-13.

Medical science had given the world new drugs which
might have assured the control of venereal diseases.
However, blacks were excluded which leads the author to
conclude that control of venereal diseases in blacks was
not strictly a medical problem.   Notes that the problem
was one of breaking down the barriers contributing to
"social sickness."   Numerous studies, as the article
refers to, have shown that social ills existed to a
greater extent among lower income people.   A study
revealed a venereal disease rate of 34.6 percent per
1000 population among individuals with incomes less than
$1,000 annually.   For blacks, the venereal disease
problem was particularly acute.   Surveys and studies
show syphilis among blacks to be "six times higher than
among whites."   Selective service reports show over 14
times as much syphilis among blacks than among whites.
Concludes that blacks have to overcome their illiteracy
to help combat the problem because America is not.

094.   Bent, M. J.   "Health Education Programs of Government
Agencies,"   Journal of Negro Education 6 (1937):499-505.

Discusses the lack of government health programs for
blacks in the 1930s.   Argues that the mortality rates
for blacks would decrease if more and better programs
were instituted.   Blacks are not adequately represented
in the public health professions.   More blacks are
needed to run these programs.   Properly trained blacks
would be more responsive to the needs of their own race
than white health professionals.

095.   Bent, M. J.   "Nutritional Deficiency as an Etiological
Factor in Icterus Accompanying Pneumonia in the Negro,"
Southern Medical Journal 138 (11) (November 1945): 730-733.

Examines the period of 1936-38 and observes an incidence
of 67.7 percent icterus accompanying lobar pneumonia in
a group of seventy-four cases of black adults in George
W. Hubbard Hospital.   Concludes from other studies
(Christian, Elton, Bianchi, and Maugeri) that a higher
incidence of icterus accompanying pneumonia occurs more
in blacks as compared to whites.   Conducts a series of
studies on normal blacks to determine whether there is a
detectable physiological basis for this difference.
Notes that inadequate diets, particularly lacking
vitamin B complex is one factor.   Adequate quantities of
brewer's yeast added to the inadequate diet was used in
this experiment.   The experimental results parallel the
clinical observations.

096. Bent, M. J. and Greene, E. F. Rural Negro Health
(Nashville, TN: Julius Rosenwald Fund, 1937).

A report submitted to the Joint Health Education
Committee regarding the mortality rates of blacks as
compared to whites in the rural South. The report is
based on a 5 year experiment in health education in the
State of Tennessee. The report was conducted as a
result of inequalities in morbidity and mortality rates
in rural black schools and communities, and sought to
determine what racial differences if any, existed in
mortality rates in the State of Tennessee and what could
be done to reduce these excessive rates. The first such
study of mortality trends in the State of Tennessee was
conducted by Dr. Elbridge Sibley. Sibley is credited
with being one of the first to note the mortality
differences between blacks and whites in the rural
South. Sibley's study led to a second investigation to
determine the etiology of such variances. This second
study examined such variables as health knowledge, home
environment, and school environment. As a result of the
second study, specific recommendations were made to the
Joint Health Committee. These recommendations were
considered the second part of the experiment with the
third part revolving around effective decreases in
mortality rates. These recommendations included such
conditions as modernize school buildings to bring them
in accord with present day standards of hygiene and
sanitation, incorporation of health education programs,
and place in the hands of school teachers free health
literature and employ full time field workers. The
Rural Negro Health concluded its experiment with the
assumption that marked differences in the mortality and
morbidity rate of blacks as compared to whites was due
not to biological factors but social and economic
factors. It concluded that health programs should be
established to educate the black as to how best to
protect himself from disease. The report also resulted
in a course of study being recommended for the training
of teachers in Health Education.

097. "Better Health for Negroes Aim of Parish Units,"
National Negro Health News 2 (July - September 1947): 12.

The Winn-Jackson Parish Health Unit promotes community
organization for better health among blacks of Winn
Parish, LA. This project involved many community groups
with the single purpose to improve the health
environment of blacks. The first phase involved the
clean-up program. This portion emphasized picking up
trash in black neighborhoods and surrounding areas and a
move to improve water sewage. Several movies were shown
on how to practice social hygiene. The second phase
involved a clinic held for all crippled children in Winn
Parish. Free examinations were offered to all crippled
children.

098.   Bevis, W. M.   "Psychological Traits of the Southern
Negro with Observations as to Some of His Psychoses,"
American Journal of Psychiatry 78 (July 1921/22): 76-78.

Examines certain phylogenetic traits of character,
habit, and behavior in the black race. Discusses their
importance to certain psychoses that are more frequently
seen in blacks. Concludes that: (1) the Southern black
has certain psychological traits that are reflected in
these psychoses; (2) motion, rhythm, music and
excitement make up a large part of the life of this
race; (3) most of the race lives in the care free or
here now, and are limited to recall or profit by
experiences of the past; (4) of all the fears,
superstitious ideas are most common; (5) suicide is
infrequent in the black race; and (6) mechanistic
classification of the psychoses of this race show that
nearly all are disassociation, compensatory of
repression types.

099.   Blackman, N.   "The Problem of Military Delinquency: A
Statistical Study of 2,142 General Prisoners," Journal of
Clinical Psychopathology and Psychotherapy 8 (1947): 849-861.

The occurrence of an "alcoholic determinant" and of
"chronic alcoholism" among 2,142 general prisoners in a
disciplinary barrack of the United States Army is
discussed. The social insecurity of blacks is confirmed
by the predominance of single men, broken homes and
poorer social integration. The lower incidence of
alcohol determinants and nomadism among blacks might be
due to the great social punishment they are exposed to
when they are either alcoholic or nomadic.

100.   Blanton, Wyndham B.   "Plantation Medicine," Medicine in
Virginia in the Eighteenth Century (Richmond, VA: 1931):
153-177.

This chapter provides a resume of the health of blacks
from the time they were brought from Africa to America,
the diseases that afflicted them, and the care bestowed
on them by their masters. The chapter attempts to
describe statistically that in 1850 the life expectancy
of the adult was about the same for both blacks and
whites. The life expectancy of the twenty-year-old
white was about 23-72, and for the black 22-70.

101.   Bloch, R. G., Tucker, W. B., and Bryant, J. E.
"Roentologic Group Examination for Pulmonary Tuberculosis,"
The Journal of the American Medical Association 115 (1940):
1866-1873.

A study of 9,000 blacks in the Chicago area for
determination of tuberculosis cases by routine
fluoroscopy of the chest. In addition to lung diseases,
the technique also revealed other nonpulmonary diseases
in the chest. Tables include record forms, clinical
classification of cases found by x-ray exams, incidence
of positive exams, age distribution and influence of

various factors on incidence of pulmonary disease. Also
given are pictures of actual x-rays of lungs with signs
of tuberculosis.

102. Blount, George W.   "The Drama of a Negro Health
Clinic," Southern Workman 62 (February 1933): 65-76.

Examines the efforts being made by blacks to improve the
efficiency and health conditions at the health clinic
serving their population in Chester and Delaware
Counties, Pennsylvania. Most of the article places
emphasis on the incidence of tuberculosis. Despite
institutional care being recommended for these patients,
there are not enough beds to go around. A clinic is
held every Tuesday, with an average of five new
patients. The nurse at the clinic begins her duties
earlier than the physician. As the patients arrive, she
will perform her routine duties, i.e. take their
temperature, pulse, respiration, and weight. The
article points out that blacks are badly in need of
increased hospital and clinical advantages.
Tuberculosis alone is not only influenced by social life
conditions, but in turn, reacts upon those conditions in
a most destructive way.

103. Boas, Ernst P.   "The Cost of Medical Care as a Factor
in the Availability of Health Facilities for Negroes,"
Journal of Negro Education 18 (Summer 1949):333-9.

Postulates that medical care has become a commodity
instead of a personal health and social service. Blacks
are unable to afford insurance and this in turn makes
medical care unaffordable for them. Concludes by
pointing out that the federal government is in a better
position than the states to render affordable medical
care to all citizens.

104. Boland, Frank K., "Morsus Humanus, Sixty Cases of Human
Bites in Negroes," Journal of American Medical Association
116 (January-May 1941):   127-130.

Examines the trauma caused by human teeth (Morsus
Humanus) by black assailants and to black victims.
Focuses on three factors involved in the destructive and
dangerous lesions which result from apparently mild
trauma and the pathological processes that take place in
the tendon sheaths, joints, and facial plances that are
caused by human bites. Special attention is devoted to
the Blue-gummed black patient because it has been
believed such a bite from a Blue-gum is deadly.
Concludes that the bite of the Blue-gummed black is no
more dangerous than the bite of any other member of the
race who's gums are not blue.

105. Bousfield, M. O.   "Reaching the Negro Community,"
American Journal of Public Health 24 (March 1934):209-215.

Outlines an approach to get health programs into the
black community. In the typical industrial city, blacks

are quartered along railroads or dirty streams.
Overcrowding is a certain result. There is a lack of
sunshine, fresh air, cleanliness, play space, and normal
recreation. Though it is essential, it is unpopular to
spend money on black health. The health program should
consist of two visits by the black patient. The first
visit will entail taking a medical history, urine
sample, and blood test. On the second visit, the
patient is advised of his condition, but no treatment is
rendered.

106. Bousfield, M. O. "An Account of Physicians of Color in
the United States," Bulletin of the History of Medicine 17
(1945):61-84.

A paper presented before the New York Society for
Medical History in February, 1944. Examines three
periods of colored physicians in the United States: the
slavery years, 1865 to 1930, and 1930 to the time of the
article. Discusses a number of black physicians who
became famous during each of these time periods and
lists the names of doctors that graduated from various
institutions during the second period. Also discusses
black physicians that served throughout history in the
military as well as those that provided service through
public service agencies. Concludes by addressing the
need for black medical schools and facilities.

107. Bousfield, M. O. "The Adventure of Public Health
Nursing," Southern Workman 61 (January 1932): 33-37.

Describes the activities of public health nursing in
East Carroll Parish, Louisiana where 75 percent of the
population is black and almost half of the 9,000 tenant
farmers needed assistance from the local Red Cross
chapter during early 1931. The efforts of the nurses
were instrumental in inoculating the residents with
typhoid fever shots and that there were only 2 typhoid
deaths. They also provided midwife instruction. Points
out how these nurses are constantly busy whether it be
conducting classes or providing vaccinations. According
to the author, the success of this nursing program is
largely attributable to the Julius Rosenwald Fund and
the National Negro Health Movement.

108. Bousfield, M. O. "The Negro Home and The Health
Education Program," Journal of Negro Education 6 (1937):
513-518.

Addresses the problems involved in health education,
first noting that there are many thousands of public
health workers and over one million school teachers.
Thus, he says there are enough health officials and
enough teachers, but the problem is that medical
personnel do not know how to teach and the teachers do
not know enough about health to teach it effectively.
Briefly discusses the joint effort of the American
Medical Association and National Educational Association
to address this problem. Argues that much of the health

education aimed at young school children is wasted and that one must reach into the home and train adults in health. Any school program that is going to be successful must reach the home environment. Discusses the requirements for such a program arguing that federal agencies must play a leadership role in the effort. Concludes with a brief discussion of the role of the teacher in this overall effort and emphasizes the need to extend the program into the home and the need for federal leadership.

109. Bowcock, Harold M. "Diabetes Mellitus in the Negroes: A Study of One Hundred Consecutive Cases," Annals of Internal Medicine 6 (1932/33): 843-844.

A study of one hundred cases of diabetes mellitus occurring in the colored race. The disease was found to occur in pure blacks as well as mulattoes. The sex incidence was predominately female. In a large majority of the cases the appearance of the disease has been preceded by marked obesity in the female patients. The disease is usually mild and the greatest handicap to adequate control is poor cooperation due to poverty and the lack of intelligence. The same complications appear in the black and the white diabetic. Successful results can be obtained in colored patients after "painstaking instruction, in the general principles of diet, insulin, and the technique of testing urine for sugar. The results are promising when viewed from an economic standpoint, although they are far from ideal."

110. Brailey, Miriam E. "Prognosis in White and Colored Tuberculous Children According to Initial Chest X-ray Findings," American Journal of Public Health 33 (April 1943):343-346.

Discusses the extent of chest lesions revealed at initial x-ray examinations in a group of 1,148 tuberculous children whose infection was discovered prior to 15 years of age, and who have been followed for varying periods of time in a study of their mortality from tuberculosis. Exposure from the community at large appears to account for infection in a somewhat larger proportion of black infants. So far as duration of household contact could be estimated, black children had less exposure than white children, but black children were treated at facilities less than whites. Both races were turned down for treatment when the tuberculosis had reached advanced stages.

111. Branche, G. C. "Tryparsamide Therapy of Neurosyphilis in Negroes," Venereal Disease Information 12 (June 20, 1931): 283-384.

According to the author, marked physical and mental improvement followed the use of tryparsamide as the treatment for neurosyphilitic blacks. The treatment was given to 29 hospital patients. The various cases resulting from neurosyphilis were 1 case of tabes dorsalis, 10 cases of cerebrospinal syphilis, and paralysis. The neurologic signs remained unchanged after the exposure to tryparsamide except for some improvements in the speech defect and tremors. The treatment of blacks with tryparsamide was highly recommended "because of Negroes apparent immunity to malaria."

112. Breidenbach, Jr., W. C. and Palmer, D. M. "Thromboangiitis Obliterans in the Negro: Report of a Case and Review of the Literature," American Heart Journal 33 (6) (June 1947): 849-855.

A case of thromboangiitis obliterans occurring in a black is described. A review of all previous reports of this uncommon combination is presented. Viewpoints on what constitutes adequate pathologic evidence of this condition are considered and treatment is discussed in relation to the sequence of pathologic changes.

113. Brenman, Margaret. "Urban Lower-Class Negro Girls," Psychiatry 6 (3) (August 1943): 307-324.

Some observations on a group of lower-class urban black girls. The data were gathered in two ways: by adopting the role of a "participant observer" and by the use of a modified clinical interview. Includes a discussion of the reaction of the lower-class black girl to her minority-group membership, inter-racial attitudes, and sexual behaviors and morality standards. The feelings and behavior of the girls in this group cannot be understood except in terms of the attempted incorporation of the values of majority society and the realistic barriers opposing this process, barriers peculiar to minority-groups. The most important conclusion suggested is that the adjustment of a member of a minority-group is always conditioned by the interplay of the normal strivings of the person and the psychological strength of the barriers to the "forbidden areas."

114. Brinton, Hugh P. "Regional Variation in Disabling Sickness Among a Group of Negro Male Railroad Employees," Journal of Social Forces 20 (December 1941): 264-270.

Discusses differences in the frequency and duration of disabling sickness among black male railroad employees using sick benefit organization records. Apparently, blacks have a slightly higher rate of sickness and nonindustrial injuries in the South than the North. Based on the observations conducted, the author concludes that there is no evidence that Northern conditions produce a greater frequency of disabilities that lasted eight days or longer.

115. Brittain, Rollo H., "New Light on the Relation of Housing to Health," American Journal of Public Health 32 (February 1943): 193-195.

A discussion on public health and the importance of environment. Argues that good housing is a right of every citizen including blacks and presents statistical data on diseases and health problems and tries to show a correlation between housing and health factors. Concludes that bad housing is a result of economic conditions for blacks; bad health is another symptom.

116. Britten, Rollo H. "The National Health Survey: Receipt of Medical Services in Different Urban Population Groups," Public Health Reports 55 (November 29, 1940): 2199-2224.

A summary of the data reported in the National Health Survey regarding the receipt of medical care. Factors included in the discussion as having an important relation to the receipt of medical services are size of city, economic status, age, diagnosis and race. Concludes that the highest illness rates and least amount of medical care were found in groups having the lowest economic status, that is mainly blacks and the poor. Extensive statistical data include more than 20 figures and tables.

117. Brodie, Jessie B. "Opportunities for Nutritional Research in the South", Journal of the American Dietetic Association 11 (3) (September 1935):217-220.

Argues that the high concentration of blacks in the South affords many research possibilities. "Foods such as turnip greens, mustard greens, collards, 'polk', okra, sweet potato, white corn, black-eyed peas, and hominy grits are consumed in massive amounts." Thus, the effects of such consumption may be studied in great detail. Cooking methods, effect of flavor, digestibility, and nutritive value of these foods are cited as possible research topics. And since these studies would look at nutritional value of several typically 'black' food items, benefits could be vast for the black communities.

118. Brown, Roscoe C. "The Health Education Programs of Government and Voluntary Agencies," Journal of Negro Education 18 (1949): 377-387.

The author opens with a description of the health education programs of several government health agencies, including the Public Health Service, the Office of Education, the Extension Service of the Department of Agriculture, departments of health at the state and local levels, and also voluntary health agencies. Provides a fairly detailed discussion of the activities of each of these agencies and organizations. Also discusses other organizations working for the general welfare of blacks in the area of health. Among these are the NAACP, National Urban League, National Council of Negro Women, and others. Discusses the activities and accomplishments of the National Negro Health Week Movement, which was founded by Booker T.

Washington in 1915. The author calls on blacks to be
conscious of the possibilities for health education.

119. Brown, Roscoe C. "The Work of the U.S. Public Health
Service with Negroes," Opportunity 1 (2) (February 1923):
12-13.

Lists and describes the activities of the United States
Public Health Service. The Service must reach the
individual person and family for both educational and
material assistance. There is special need of contact
and work with special groups by trained persons
identified with the group, who because of the definite
knowledge of the conditions and problems affecting the
group, have a favorable approach. Explains that the
United States Public Health Service has given effective
cooperation in promoting the National Negro Health Week
and in developing appreciation for the need of a
constant year-round health program to be propagated by
individual states and communities through state and
local health departments and efficient voluntary health
and social service agencies. The policy of the work
being done with the black population through
representatives of its own group is not one of isolation
or discrimination, but a policy of adaptation, whereby
the special public health needs of the country are
served through the most logical and efficient procedure.

120. Brown, Roscoe C. "The National Negro Health Week
Movement," Journal of Negro Education 6 (1937):553-64.

An account of the development of the National Negro
Health Week. This movement is an annual weekly
observance in which organizations at the national,
state, and local levels meet to discuss methods to
"improve the health of Negroes and the conditions under
which they live." A national committee provides
suggestions to the committees at the lower levels and
stimulates people to improve the sanitary conditions in
their communities. Included in the article is a typical
bulletin describing the objectives, activities, and
plans surrounding the Week. Data relating to the 1936
National Health Week is presented. For the year 1936,
in which thirty states and twenty-eight hundred
communities participated, the data reveal that 65,100
homes and lots were cleaned up, 35,015 insect and rodent
control activities were performed, and 418,000 people
attended lectures relating to black health improvement.
The conclusion provides a listing of the qualifications
of the black leaders of the National Negro Health Week.
The author was a Health Educational Specialist for the
U.S. Public Health Service.

121. Brown, W. Roderick. "New Control of Tuberculosis," The
Crisis 46 (May 1937): 139-140.

Although stimulated by the progress which has already
been made, the culmination of the greatest ambitions of
blacks will not have been accomplished until blacks have

relegated this lethal destroyer (tuberculosis) of human happiness to the cemetery of complete oblivion. Much more remains to be done and will be accomplished if only those engaged in this worthy battle are given the heartly cooperation of their patients, adequate opportunity for clinical study, suitable material for scientific research and the needed financial assistance.

122. Bryant, Bertha. "Five Years in a Negro Health Program," Public Health Nursing 27 (June 1935): 324-326.

In 1930, the Delaware County Tuberculosis Association saw the need to address the widespread mortalities associated with Tuberculosis. However, those in charge felt that such a program could only be effective if blacks were involved. Blacks are experiencing mortality rates of 2 to 1 as compared to whites. As a result, a group of the 35 most influential blacks were assembled and the public health program was initiated. The plan included providing for a black health clinic along with a black physician and all black employees. The program called not only for immediate medical attention, but attempted to combat chronic health problems in the black community. The public health nurse was responsible for interviewing all new patients and responding to black social health problems. Supervision is provided to teach blacks proper sanitation, diets, and personal hygiene.

123. "Bulletin on Mortality Among Negroes," Journal of the American Medical Association 90 (3) (January 21, 1928):214.

An announcement of the Bulletin Number 174 issued by the U.S. Health Service summarizing data published annually by the Census Bureau concerning mortality among blacks. Attention is called to the diseases which are more of a menace to blacks than to whites. Tables showing the distribution of the black population in the United States, mortality from important causes by age and color, and the trend of mortality in Baltimore, Charleston and New Orleans for the period 1870-1923 are presented.

124. Burch, George and Winson, Travis. "Sickle-Cell Anemia: A Great Masquerader," Journal of the American Medical Association 129 (12) (November 17, 1945):793-794.

Begins by comparing sickle cell anemia to the disease syphilis. The similarity is mentioned because both diseases are so subtle as to not even enter a physician's mind during diagnosis. Thus because of this problem, it is necessary to study all black patients for sickle cell. Discusses two methods which lend themselves well to the routine testing of black patients for sickle cell anemia. The two methods are: the tourniquet technique and the carbon dioxide technique. Of the 612 blacks tested, 27 cases of active sickle cell were found.

125. Burney, L. E. "Control of Syphilis in a Southern Rural Area," American Journal of Public Health 29 (September 1939):1006-14.

Discusses a program enacted in Georgia to control syphilis in the rural black. A mobile clinic was used as the examining facility. It was able to cover a large amount of territory and travel to the deep woods where many blacks live. House-to-house canvassing for blood testing was also done. Concludes that blacks need to be taught the facts about syphilis through movies, simple literature, black ministers, and school teachers. A successful follow-up worker is essential in the treatment of those blacks who have already contracted the disease.

126. Butterworth, John B. "Hereditary Spherocytic Anemia in the Negro," Journal of the American Medical Association 144 (16) (December 16, 1950): 1404-1405.

Presents a study of four generations of blacks (12), two of whom (both women) had hereditary spherocytic anemia. Splenectomy was performed on one and the blood values returned to normal. Concludes that a simple single gene, dominant-recessive relation is not an explanation for the disease. Spherocytic anemia in blacks is due to a multiple of factors. Also discusses the high incidence of disease in the female.

127. By a Group of Students at Washington Jr. High School, Nashville, Tennessee. "What People Really Know About Tuberculosis," Opportunity 20 (12) (December 1942): 363-364.

This essay, by the students of the Washington Junior High School from Nashville, Tennessee, won first prize of $50.00 and a gold medal offered to high school students in the Annual Negro Essay Contest conducted by the National Tuberculosis Association. It was read at the Southern Tuberculosis Conference held in Memphis, Tennessee, on October 7, by Pearl May Gore, one of the students who participated in the project. The students confined their discussion to four topics: (1) What people know about tuberculosis; (2) What people do not know about tuberculosis; (3) What facts students consider the most important; and (4) What needs to be done about it. Points out several facts which should be known and applied: Tuberculosis is caused by a germ, the tubercle bacillus, which usually lodges in the lung, but may occur in other parts of the body. Tuberculosis is not inherited. Tuberculosis often exists without the presence of symptoms. Tuberculosis is curable. Through this survey and discussion, it was concluded that this information would increase general knowledge about tuberculosis, reduce, and in time eradicate this disease.

128. Caldwell, Helen S., "Freedom From Disease a Challenge to Education," National Negro Health News 15 (1) (January-March 1947):5-6.

Urges that emphasis on the improvement of black health conditions be placed on education of the individual, the family and the community. In a brief summary of the history of high black morbidity and mortality rates, cites primary early causes as hard labor, lack of proper natal care, sexual promiscuity and unchecked communicable disease. Points out primary causes of high black mortality as chronic heart disease, nephritis, tuberculosis, and maternal and infant mortality. Suggests that since economic and social factors and psychological adjustment to them are directly related, the solution lies in health education. Concludes that all institutions of learning (including churches and civic organizations) bear the responsibility for health education in the black community. Describes the National Negro Health Week Movement as an example of positive community involvement.

129. Callis, H. A. "The Need and Training of Negro Physicians," Journal of Negro Education (1936):32-41.

Notes that there are less than 4,000 black physicians for 12 million blacks. For the past 20 years there has been no substantial gain in the number of black physicians. Some 60 percent of the present number possess poor clinical and hospital facilities. The public health, social and economic problems which the black physician faces, are more intense than those for the country as a whole. The black physician is handicapped and ostracized in all his professional opportunities for development and service. Nevertheless, the black physician has been one of the strongest factors in the advancement of blacks in America.

130. Callis, H. A. "The Incidence of Physical Defects in Negro Adults," The Journal of Negro Education 6 (July 1937): 396-398.

Examines the commonly held notion that there is a higher incidence of physical defects among blacks which is assumed to be the result of genetic deficiency of the race. Concludes that there exists little evidence or factual data on the incidence of physical defects in blacks, that inherited defects probably occur with the same mathematical infrequency in blacks as they do in all other humans, and that any data on physical defects among blacks must be analyzed within the context of nutritional, occupational and economic factors.

131. Callis, H. A. "Immediate Health Problems: Need of Opportunities for Continuous Training of the Negro Physician." National Negro Health News 2 (3) (1934): 20.

Notes that better training of black physicians is very important and argues for increased facilities for hospital and clinic opportunities as well as for postgraduate instruction. These activities would improve health conditions, help the community

economically, and should be applied throughout the
nation. With more cooperation between the two major
racial groups, plans could be developed whereby the
black physician would be given the opportunity for
continuous, local training, and a great deal could be
accomplished in a few years toward the improvement of
black health.

132. Callis, H. A. "Leading Causes of Death Among Negroes:
the Degenerative Diseases." Journal of Negro Education 18
(Summer 1949): 235-239.

     Examines degenerative diseases and length of life of
     blacks. After an examination of standardized death
     rates in 1940 concludes that blacks have a 71 percent
     higher chance of dying from degenerative diseases than
     whites. Yet, this was an improvement over the 1930
     figure of 81 percent. Also concludes that aging
     increases significance of degenerative diseases and that
     longevity of life from other diseases for blacks has
     increased.

133. Campagna, Maurice. "Peptic Ulcers in the Negro," New
Orleans Medical and Surgical Journal 92 (December
1939):366-368.

     A paper read before the Louisiana Medical Society in
     April of 1939. Discusses the lack of attention given to
     peptic ulcers in blacks. Reports findings of a study in
     which 37 percent of 300 autopsy cases revealed peptic
     ulcers as the cause of death. Concludes that out of the
     300 cases, only 2 tested syphilis positive which
     disputed the belief that syphilis played an active part
     in a great majority of stomach disorders in blacks.

134. Carley, Paul S. and Wenger, O. C. "The Prevalence of
Syphilis in Apparently Healthy Negroes in Mississippi,"
Journal of the American Medical Association 94 (23) (June 7,
1930):1826-1829.

     A study in Mississippi in three selected rural counties
     where the ratio of blacks to whites is at least 5:1. Of
     7,228 blood samples above the age of nine, 19.3 percent
     of the males and 18.0 percent of the females were
     positive. Argues that the findings are an underestimate
     of the actual rate in the group. Concludes that
     "syphilis is probably the major public health problem
     among rural Mississippi negroes today."

135. Carter, Elmer A. "Infant Mortality in New York,"
Opportunity 9 (4) (April 1931): 105.

     Cites data published by the New York City Department of
     Health which strengthens the argument by competent and
     authentic authorities that the high death rate among
     blacks is less a matter of race than a matter of proper
     surroundings, recreational opportunity, sanitary
     housing, health education, and adequate income. In 1929
     the infant mortality rate for black residents in New

York was 101 per thousand, the lowest probably in
history. It was still nearly twice as high as the
infant mortality rate for the white population, but the
figures for the black rate by area show that in many
cases it is less than the rate for white residents of
the same areas. Reiterates that if blacks could sustain
within the next decade the economic progress which has
been attained since the World War, there can be little
doubt that in cities of the North especially, their
mortality rate will steadily decrease as their span of
life increases.

136. Carter, Elmer A. "Health Statistics," Opportunity 10
(8) (August 1932): 239.

An editorial which suggests that there exists the
assumption that blacks have a peculiar susceptibility to
pulmonary diseases. As a result, many individuals and
communities accept the high morbidity and mortality rate
of blacks as inevitable and are reluctant to sponsor or
inaugurate adequate programs for health improvement.
Presents a disturbing statement found in a bulletin from
the Department of Health in the City of New York which
reads as follows: "It will be seen that the Central
Harlem Health District as a whole has the highest number
of new cases of tuberculosis. This is usually explained
by the very large Negro population among whom
tuberculosis is very pervalent." However, a study of a
poor white section as compared with a black section of
the better class in the City of Cincinnati revealed the
fact that the mortality rate from tuberculosis for
whites was 673 per 100,000 and for blacks, the rate was
0. Concludes by observing how clear it is that we must
not be so ready to explain high morbidity rates by the
racial composition of a population. Social and economic
conditions are the chief deciding factors.

137. Carter, Elmer A. "Racial Prejudice in the Medical
Profession," Opportunity 12 (10) (October 1934): 295.

In the Directory of Physicians and Surgeons for the year
1933 a strange procedure is inaugurated (apparently with
the approval of the American Medical Association) which
is an indefensible example of racial discrimination.
All black physicians and surgeons therein are designated
by race, for unknown reasons, unless it is to imply a
racial inferiority which cannot be established otherwise
than by a subtle appeal to existing racial prejudices.
Physicians of other races are listed but their racial
deviation is omitted. Recognizes the distinguished
contributions of Dr. Louis T. Wright, a black whose
surgical technique and practice surely cannot be
designated by race or color. The action of the editors
of the Directory of Physicians and Surgeons in isolating
black members of the profession is more than an
indication of petty racial preduice; it is a sad
reflection on their intellectual integrity. In the
realm of science, if nowhere else, there can be no
racial standards.

138. "Cause of Death," Journal of the American Medical Association 87 (17) (October 23, 1926):1399.

A medical note report of a study by the Maryland State Department of Health of the causes of death in the white and black races in the state during the past three years. The leading causes of deaths are, for whites, Heart Disease; Bright's Disease; Cerebral Hemorrhage; Cancer; and, Tuberculosis. For blacks, Tuberculosis; Heart Disease; Cerebral Hemorrhage; Bright's Disease; and, Diarrhea and Enteritis.

139. Chinn, May E. "Cancer and The Negro," Opportunity 15 (February 1937):51-53.

Presents cancer data on the American black. Compares the frequency of various types of cancer in black men and women and white men and women. Addresses the early signs of cancer, treatment of cancer, how to obtain treatment, curability of cancer and prevention of cancer. Concludes that blacks appear to be as susceptible to cancer as whites.

140. Chivers, Walter R. "Northward Migration and the Health of Negroes," The Journal of Negro Education 8 (January 1939):34-43.

Surveys the significant differences in environment resulting from migrations of blacks from the rural South to the urban North and various areas of health among blacks affected by these changes in environment. Citing numerous studies of the health of blacks in various parts of the country, discusses the effects of this migration on tuberculosis, syphilis, and psychopathic sequelae. The increased incidence of these diseases can be attributed to the changes in environment due to migration. Family units are frequently broken up due to loss of a parent (usually the father) during migration. Housing in large black ghettoes in urban areas is frequently worse than that in rural areas. The increased availability of medical services and means for evaluating mortality and morbidity may also account for the increased number of cases 'reported' or discovered. The mass migrations of blacks has created a negative attitude toward them which has affected their socialization and so their treatment. The lack of recreational facilities for blacks in urban areas has contributed to an increase in crime (hence homicide) among blacks. And finally, migration to the industrial North has increased both the desire for more among blacks and at the same time the stress of being unable to achieve this goal. The resulting frustration has caused an increase in black psychopathic behavior such as suicide. Ultimately, the author places much of the blame for blacks' seeming inability to adjust to the indifferent attitude of the white race.

141. Clark, Taliaferro. "The Negro Tuberculosis Problem,"
Transactions of the Twenty-eighth Annual Meeting of the
National Tuberculosis Association (1932).

>   Observes that blacks should be provided more free clinic
>   and hospital care, better insanitary conditions and
>   living environment to lower the tuberculosis mortality
>   rates among them. Also recommend actions needed to help
>   blacks in fighting diseases. (1) Increasing attention
>   to the dissemination of information with regard to the
>   dangers of tuberculosis, the necessity for prompt care
>   and attention, including medical advice and emphasis on
>   the hope of recovery. (2) The training and employment
>   of black public health nurses for tuberculosis work
>   among members of their own race. (3) Better training of
>   black medical students in the diagnosis and management
>   of tuberculosis, and provision of facilities and
>   opportunity for clinical study by practicing black
>   physicians. (4) The assumption of responsiblity by the
>   State and community for the provision of (a) more
>   adequate dispensaries and follow-up service for the
>   diagnosis of cases and supervision of the ambulant sick;
>   (b) increased hospitalization of advanced cases in order
>   to limit the spread of infection; (c) sanatoria for
>   patients who have hope of arrest.

142. Clark, Taliaferro, Heller, J R., Vonderhehr, R. A. and
Wenger, O. C. "Untreated Syphilis in the Negro Male: A
Comparative Study of Treated and Untreated Cases," Journal of
the American Medical Association 107 (11) (September 12,
1936): 856-860.

>   A study of 399 males with syphilis who had never
>   received treatment, 201 nonsyphilis black males and 275
>   black males who had received treatment during the first
>   two years of having the disease. Concludes that the
>   cardiovascular system is very commonly involved in the
>   late syphilitic process and the death rate of black
>   males that are untreated is far higher than that of the
>   non-syphilitic groups.

143. Cobb, W. M. "Your Nose Won't Tell," Crisis 45 (10)
(October 1938):332, 336.

>   Refutes the statement of Victor Heiser that the split
>   cartilege in the nose is the true test of black blood.
>   Points out anatomical and anthropological studies which
>   indicate "that no cartilege is known to split in any
>   human nose; and the the presence or absence of the
>   median septal or apical sulcus is not a criterion for
>   Negro blood."

144. Cobb, W. M. "Education in Human Biology: An Essential
for the Present and the Future," Journal of Negro History 28
(2) (April 1943): 119-155.

>   Main subject matter is physical anthropology - human
>   variation and attendant conditions. Common to all
>   humans are the variables: age, sex, race, and body type.

The negroid pigmentation is not fully developed until
some days after birth, but in the white person, a
tendency to the broadening of the features and frizzling
of the hair sets in the progressive years. Argues that
the general public needs to be educated in human
biology, since popular misinterpretation of the
importance of race has caused more social harm than any
of the other variables. But in biological perspective,
race has little importance for social majority -
minority relationships. Presents diagrams representing
the evolution of man in the "Distinctive Features of the
Higher Primates" and contends that characteristics used
as racial criteria have taxonomic value rather than
survival value, then goes on to dispel some rumors. Two
features based on fallacious notions, namely, the
assertion that the possession of a one-piece cartilage
in the nose was a reliable test of black blood, since
all other races had a split cartilage; and the assertion
that the success of the black track field stars was due
to a longer heel bone than that of a white are
dissipated. Such examples that blacks are biologically
different than other races imply qualities to which race
has no organic relation. Consequently, there is nothing
unnatural or mysterious in the mixing of races.
Concludes that social problems cannot be solved unless
they are first understood.

145. Cobb, W. M. "Removing Our Health Burden," Crisis 53
(9) (September 1946):268-270, 282-283.

Encourages the passage of a national Health Bill.
Advocates the enactment of national legislation in order
to safeguard adequate medical care for all citizens.
Observes that "it cannot be overemphasized, however,
that health is not a racial problem, that the health
conditions of Negroes are largely a reflection of their
socio-economic circumstances, and that poor health in
any segment of the population is a hazard to the nation
as a whole." Discusses why the N.A.A.C.P. became
involved in securing equal medical care for blacks.
"The N.A.A.C.P. has two chief points of interest in the
profile of black health; first, that the excess Negro
mortality and concomitant morbidity are due to
preventable causes, and, second, that as improvements
are achieved, the Negro generally lags behind the white,
indicating that he does not share as rapidly or as fully
in the application of medical advances." Most of the
diseases which cause high mortality in blacks are the
result of "low economic conditions, overcrowding, poor
nutrition, bad sanitation and lack of medical care."
For this reason, argues that improvements in the
standard of living of blacks will also improve their
health. The N.A.A.C.P. supports the national
legislation, since it would improve black health as it
improves the nation's health.

146. Cobb, W. M. "Medical Care and the Plight of the
Negro," Crisis 54 (7) (June 1947):201-211.

Argues that blacks have not partaken of the advances in
the field of medicine and that both black doctors and
patients have been the victims of a segregated system in
education and medical facilities. States that "keystone
in the bad health conditions of the Negro, is his
excessive mortality, his high incidence in venereal
diseases, his lack of hospital facilities, and the
inadequate number of Negro physicians in the Negro
medical ghetto." Points out that segregated schools and
medical facilities have hampered improvement of health
in blacks and that the problem can only be solved by
making medical schools more accessible to blacks. With
an increasing number of black physicians and nurses, the
health of blacks will improve as the health of the
country improves. Also notes that black hospitals
cannot solve the health plight of blacks if the staff of
these hospitals do not receive the same educational
opportunities as their white counterparts.

147. Cobb, W. M. "Progress and Portents for the Negro in
Medicine," Crisis 55 (4) (April 1948):107-122, 125-126.

Argues that the history of blacks in medicine in the
United States is one of continuous struggle.
Segregation in professional schools and discrimination
in medical facilities have allowed a great lag in black
health. Concludes that the greatest obstacle to good
health care for blacks is the accessibility of health
care facilities both in training and treatment.

148. Cobb, W. M. "Special Problems in the Provision of
Medical Services for Negroes," Journal of Negro Education 18
(Summer 1949):340-5.

Discusses problems faced by the black medical community.
Among the difficulties cited are philosophic divergence,
factual ignorance, and segregation. Both black and
white physicians sometimes profit from segregation.
There are also indirect pressures. This is seen when
black physicians are influenced by white members of
certain boards.

149. Cohen, A. "Gout in a Negro Family," American Journal
of Medicine 4 (6) (June 1948): 911-915.

Discusses two of three black brothers who have gout.
There is very little medical literature on the incidence
of gout among blacks. The black male, J. A., born in
South Carolina in 1929, to a poor family, could afford
only ordinary diet. The disease caused swelling pains
in the bone joints of the body. The patient has had
five attacks since the age of twelve and was once
hospitalized for nineteen days, his longest stay. Fever
therapy, baking and massage, as well as the other forms
of therapy ordinarily prescribed for arthritis were
given by the hospital. Younger brother, P. A. had the
same problem and had been also attacked by the disease
several times since the age of twelve. Suggests that
one would not have a recurrent attack of acute gout wit

proper regulation of the diet, abstinence of alcoholic beverages, and proper administration of colchicin.

150.   "Color and the AMA." Newsweek 32 (July 12, 1948): 46-47.

Before any physician can join the American Medical Association, one must first become a member of the medical society in his or her county. Yet in seventeen Southern states and in the District of Columbia where the county groups observe a color barrier, no black doctor has been able to join. Since membership in the AMA was necessary before a doctor can join most hospital staffs, black physicians were further handicappped in the profession. However, on May 18, 1948, the State of New York Medical Society allowed black physicians to join, but it had no effect on the guidelines set by the AMA.

151.   "Colored Children Join in the Health Game," Crisis 26 (6) (October 1923):256, 258.

Discusses the influence of health programs of public schools on the health awareness of black children. "The health program consists of object talks, illustrated stories, classroom games, simple dramatics, songs and motion pictures." The program was established by Mrs. Madalene L. Tillman, a nutrition worker on the staff of the health department of the Philadelphia Inter-State Dairy Council. Mrs. Tillman is actively involved in teaching health to black children in Philadelphia, Atlantic City, Camden, Chester, and Trenton, New Jersey public schools. "The best thing about this health program is that the children themselves take an active part in putting it across."

152.   "Colored Doctors." The Commonweal (January 12, 1934): 284.

A summary of a report issued by the Carnegie Corporation of New York stating that there were too few blacks in the medical profession. The report had its inception in an investigation of conditions at Harlem Hospital. The report noted that there were only one-fourth as many blacks in the profession as whites. Also pointed out that very few hospitals admitted black graduates in medicine to internships, and those that did were without a salary. The report called upon hospital authorities to accept well qualified black graduates for interne services.

153.   Combs, Bessie E. "Health on Wheels in Mississippi," American Journal of Nursing 41 (May 1941): 551-554.

The involvement of the Alpha Kappa Alpha sorority, which is composed of black women, in sponsoring a clinic that travels to various Mississippi rural communities to provide medical preventive therapy and health education to black residents. The clinic is comprised of all

volunteers, including doctors and nurses. The sorority
purchased all of the supplies that were needed. The
work involving the services rendered was planned by a
medical committee of the sorority, with the approval of
the United States Public Health Service. The clinics
were established in weatherbeaten schools and churches.
The sorority went to great lengths to promote the
clinics and make them as attractive as possible. For
instance, large posters dealing with health and hygiene
were placed about the room where the services were being
performed.

154. "Conference on Negro Health Work," American Journal of
Public Health 16 (Spring 1926):31.

An important meeting was held at the Office of the
Surgeon General for the purpose of furthering health
work among the members of the colored race. A new
slogan, "More National Negro Health Work" was adopted by
the council and plans for the revision of the literature
used in connection with the program was agreed upon.
Particular emphasis was given to the importance of the
cooperation of state and local authorities in this
movement and also on the better understanding on the
part of the public that the negro health week is only
the beginning.

155. "Conference with Negro Leaders on Wartime Problems in
Venereal Disease Control," Journal of Social Hygiene 30 (2)
(February 1944): 76-79.

A conference which grew out of governmental and
voluntary discussions of what could be done at federal,
state, and local levels to reduce the spread of venereal
disease as a threatening handicap to black health and
efficiency. The three main points of discussion are:
(1) the prevalence and incidence of venereal disease
among blacks and problems involved in the control
program; (2) the role that blacks play in voluntary
organizations at a national, state, and local level to
solve this problem; and (3) the assistance that these
voluntary groups will need from public and private
agencies at all three levels. Points out that the
experiences of blacks with communicable diseases have
been similar to that of white people; however, the
social and economic conditions of blacks makes it
possible for the disease to manifest itself more
ferociously in them. Concludes that blacks cannot solve
this problem alone, the support and action of the
community as a whole is needed.

156. "Congress of Colored Parents and Teachers at Kansas
City, Kansas." National Negro Health News 15 (2) (1947): 22.

The National Congress of Colored Parents and Teachers
held its Founders Session in Kansas City, Kansas, June
15-17, 1947. Among the special features of this meeting
was a panel discussion on Health of the Negro Child.
Emphasis throughout the session of the Congress was on

the responsibility of the home, school and community for better care and training of children during their formative and developmental years. Physical and mental health were recognized as essentials for a wholesome, integrated personality that will give the child self-sufficiency to meet their problems and opportunities in later years.

157. Conn, John W., and Matthews, P. "Addison's Disease in the Negro", Journal of the Medical Sciences 212 (October 1946): 404.

Since 1907, only 21 cases of Addison's Disease had been reported in blacks (up to 1948). In 1948 five new cases in blacks were reported from the University of Michigan. Nausea, vomiting, loss of weight, asthenia, and pigmentation are symptoms of Addison's. Pigmentation is usually the key factor in the diagnosis of Addison's Disease. Since this was difficult to diagnose in blacks, the disease was not accounted for in the black population unless the patient told the doctor the specific symptoms.

158. Cooper, Chauncey I. "The Present Status of the Negro in Pharmacy," The Negro History Bulletin 3 (1939/1940):35.

About 95 percent or more of the black graduates of colleges of pharmacy enter retail drugstores, where they become proprietors, managers, pharmacists, and clerks. For the period 1931-1938, there had been an average of approximately 27 black graduates a year. The most recent data indicate that there are 1,200 registered black pharmacists in the U.S. There are five towns in Georgia with black populations ranging from six to twenty-four thousand without one black-owned drugstore. The same can be said of Florida. Clearly, there is not much of an opportunity.

159. Cooper, W. M. Health Conditions Among Negroes in Virginia (Hampton Institute, Virginia, 1937).

The author points out that general health conditions found among blacks in the State of Virginia are due largely to their economic, educational, and geographical conditions rather than to the fact that blacks belong to a different race. According to outstanding studies such as those of Dr. Louis I. Dublin of the Metropolitan Life Insurance Company, one finds that the general death rate among blacks is relatively higher than among whites. Black health conditions can be greatly improved with an increase in the educational status of blacks, the economic condition of blacks, and the sanitary surroundings in which blacks live. Therefore, the problem ought to be attacked from all angles at the same time.

160. Cornely, Paul B. "Administration of Health Education and Health Supervision in Negro Colleges," American Journal of Public Health 26 (September 1936):888-896.

According to the Committee on Approval of Negro Schools,
the enrollment at black colleges has increased in the
past 20 years. It may be assumed that if this group is
made health conscious through good health education and
health supervision, they will in turn influence their
families and communities and thus help in improving the
health of blacks. It is therefore important to know the
extent and status of health education in black colleges.
However, notes that black schools suffer from inadequate
health fees, lack of coordination of the reported
practices and procedures, and lack of adequately trained
personnel.

161. Cornely, Paul B.   "Health Education Programs in Negro
Colleges," Journal of Negro Education 6 (1937): 531-537.

Summarizes the previous literature and data on health
programs in black colleges in the United States and
presents a brief description of the history of college
health programs in America. Observes that an effective
college health program involves three phases: the
hygiene and sanitation of the campus environment,
informational hygiene, and health services to students.
Reports the findings of a survey of 32 black colleges
and examined their programs in each of these three
areas. Concludes that the findings suggest that these
institutions have inadequate health programs. Offers
suggestions as to how colleges might make improvements
in their health programs.

162. Cornely, Paul B.   "Morbidity and Mortality from Scarlet
Fever in the Negro," American Journal of Public Health 29
(September 1939):999-1005.

Focuses on the lack of comparative studies on the
scarlet fever experience of the black population in the
South with that of the North, nor has this been
contrasted with that of the white population in these
two regions. The study reports survey findings from
appropriate health service personnel. The results
indicate that the differences in scarlet fever mortality
and morbidity rates between blacks and whites is
greatest in southern states, and least in northern
states. The case fatality for all ages from scarlet
fever seems to be higher for blacks in all communities
both North and South. This is particularly true in the
under-five age group.

163. Cornely, Paul B.   "Trends in Public Health Activities
Among Negroes in 96 Southern Counties During the Period
1930-1939," American Journal of Public Health 32 (October
1942):1117-24.

Survey findings of the availability of certain health
services according to race during the decade of the
1930s. The findings revealed that tuberculosis was the
first or second cause of death among Negroes. In 1930
and 1939, the availability of clinic services for white
persons was much greater than for Negroes, although the

number of deaths was greater in the latter group. In
regard to venereal disease, the Negro had available more
clinic hours per week than white persons. By 1939, the
Negro had available 63.9 clinic hours per week per
100,000 people, as compared to 26.0 for whites. A
survey was also conducted of courses and fellowships
available to Negro health personnel in 1939. Few
courses were available for Negro physicians, nurses, and
midwives. Only fifteen fellowships were granted to
Negro physicians and nurses in 1939.

164. Cornely, Paul B. "Distribution of Negro Physicians in
the United States in 1942," Journal of the American Medical
Association 124 (March 1944):826-830.

Compares a study of the distribution of black physicians
in the U.S. conducted in 1942 with an earlier one
conducted in 1932. The study revealed that there had
been a decrease in the number of black physicians during
the decade. The ratio of black physicians to the black
population was less than one fourth that of 1 to 750 for
all physicians. The South as a whole showed the lowest
ratio. Nearly all Southern states showed ratios which
were lower than the national average. Black physicians
have a tendency to concentrate in large cities.

165. Cornely, Paul B. "Health Assets And Liabilities of The
Negro." Opportunity 23 (4) (Fall 1945): 198-200.

Although the attention of this report is focused on
blacks, the author advises that there is no such entity
as a "Negro Health Problem", because the health
achievements and problems of blacks are merely
expressions of the total health situation of the
country. Reveals data that show marked progress in the
health of blacks during the last 30 or 40 years and
cites tuberculosis as a specific disease where there has
been a downward trend in the black mortality rate during
the past 35 years. Reviews various organizations and
agencies such as the United States Public Health Service
and the Children's Bureau which have contributed greatly
to the improvement of the health of blacks. Points out
that the state and local official health agencies have
the final responsibility for the health of the people
within the confines of their communities. Makes
reference to the Julius Rosenwald Fund, a major
contributor during this period to the improvement of
health for blacks. The fund provided $300,000 for the
purpose of paying a part of the salaries for six black
public nurses and to help build a new Meharry Medical
College and Hospital.

166. Cornely, Paul B. "Race Relations in A Community Health
Organization," American Journal of Public Health 36
(September 1946):36.

Examines problems facing Negroes and health care
opportunities. A community relations project supported
by the National Urban League is offered as a method in

which communities could upgrade their health services to
Negroes. A survey of six cities found that all of them
were lacking in certain basic health programs. Most of
the voluntary health agencies lacked Negro
representation on their boards and therefore were in the
position of making plans and executing programs in which
blacks were involved without the benefit of their point
of view. A change that needed to be made was the
provision for the black point of view in health care
programs. Qualified black nurses and physicians must be
given salaries commensurate with whites. Equal
facilities such as hospitals and clinics are a further
requirement.

167. Cornely, Paul B. "Polio Control--Ten Years On The
March." Opportunity 26 (3) (July-September 1948): 111-112,
119-120.

Describes how infantile paralysis or polimoyelitis has
attacked an unusually large number of persons during the
period and how it has become a major health problem
worthy of consideration. Asks, "How does the Negro fare
in his encounter with polimoyelitis?" Data show that
blacks in Detroit and Philadelphia exceed a rate of
three times that of other population groups in the
incidence of polio. It is a fact that polio can and
does strike blacks. Stresses the importance of good
community organization in controlling an epidemic
disease. Explains basic essentials in a community
control plan: (1) early discovery of cases; (2)
facilities for treatment; (3) a program of
rehabilitation; (4) health education; and (5) research
activities. The National Foundation for Infantile
Paralysis supported by the March of Dimes, through its
many chapters, has mapped out a coordinated program with
many facts designed to help in the control of this
disease. Its charter includes that direct medical
assistance will be given to those afflicted with polio
irrespective of age, race, creed, or color.

168. Cornely, Paul B. "The Nature and Extent of Health
Education Among Negroes," The Journal of Negro Education 18
(Summer 1949): 370-376.

Observes that four major problems have caused relative
failure of health education programs: (1) health
education has not been sold to legislators and policy-
makers, therefore, there exists a lack of resources; (2)
personnel in health education are not qualified and the
field lacks standards of education and competence; (3)
little research and evaluation of health education
programs have been conducted; and (4) little effort has
been made to reach large segments of the population who
have not been reached but represent large proportions of
health problems. Concludes that lack of facilities and
attitudes of white public health workers toward blacks
have caused problems in health education of blacks.

169. Council on Medical Education and Hospitals [A Report],
The Journal of the American Medical Association 115 (1940):
1461.

A report of the hearings on the George-Wagner National
Health Bill which discussed the problems of
hospitalization of blacks. Provides selected census
data of black hospital occupancy in 1939.

170. Crabtree, James A. et al. "Syphilis in a Rural Negro
Population in Tennessee," American Journal of Public Health
22 (February 1932):157-64.

A Wassermann survey of a group of black families in
Tennessee. Of a total of 2,323 people tested,
twenty-six percent were found to have syphilis. Almost
ninety percent of these individuals were between the
ages of fifteen and fifty. The estimated annual
morbidity rate for cases of acquired syphilis in Tipton
County, Tennessee is approximately 4,233 per 100,000.
The likelihood of a pregnancy resulting in either a
stillbirth or miscarriage when either parent has a
positive Wassermann is 8.2 times that of such an
occurrence when neither parent has syphilis.

171. Crabtree, James A. "Tuberculosis Studies in Tennessee:
Tuberculosis in the Negro as Related to Certain Conditions of
Environment," Journal of the American Medical Association 101
(10) (September 2, 1933):756-761.

A tuberculosis study conducted in Tennessee in 1930,
which included the entire population of the City of
Kingsport. Elements of the study included age,
cleanliness of the house, number of rooms, water supply,
disposal of excretia, consumption of milk, and income of
the wage earners. Of the 556 persons included in the
study, a total of 52 fatal and non-fatal cases were
discovered. In addition, those households where
tuberculosis was discovered were more crowded, had
larger families, milk consumption was lower, and there
was evidence of filth and untidiness in the home. The
study showed no prevalence of tuberculosis in any
occupation other than the day laborer.

172. Craig, Robert M, Schwemlein, George X., Barton, Robert
L., Bauer, Theodore J. and Bundesen, Herman H. "Penicillin
the Treatment of Early Syphilis, 429 Patients Treated with
1,200,000 units in 90 Hours," Annals of Internal Medicine 27
(1947): 225-230.

A total of 429 patients (362 Blacks and 66 whites) were
treated for darkfield positive syphilis. Each patient
received 40,000 oxford units of sodium penicillin (1.2
million total) intramuscularly every three hours for 30
doses, over a period of three and three-quarter days.
Eighty-five patients were considered treatment failures.
Concludes that the schedule of treatment appears to be
more effective than smaller amounts of penicillin either

alone, or in combination with arsenicals administered
over twice the time period.

173. Crooles, K. B. M.   "Color Blindness Among Negroes,"
Human Biology 8 (September 1936):451-458.

Discusses the genealogical tracing of color blindness in
blacks.

174. Davis, C. W.   "Health Education Programs in Negro
Colleges and Universities," Journal of Negro Education 18
(Summer 1949): 409-417.

Describes some recent movements to improve black college
health programs (e.g., formation of National Student
Health Association, American Social Hygiene Association,
various state and national conferences, etc.) and the
activities of the School-Health Coordinating Service of
North Carolina and the Conference of College Health and
P. E. Teachers to develop standards for health education
instruction. Also describes health education programs
at several black universities (e.g., Florida A & M,
State Teachers College at Montgomery, Ala. and Meharry
Medical College and Howard University). Concludes that
colleges should evaluate their programs against
standards set by the American Student Health Association
and work to achieve accreditation.

175. Davis, Michael M.   "Problems of Health Service for
Negroes," Journal of Negro Education 6 (1937):438-49.

Discusses black health care as a problem in four areas:
"medical, economic, racial, and educational." Members
of all races are more susceptible to death by such
diseases as tuberculosis when they are in the lower end
of the socioeconomic spectrum. Yet, poor areas of the
country (particularly the South) lack the resources to
better their people economically or medically. The
racial policies of segregation in regard to medical
facilities exacerbate the problem for blacks. Health
education and health care are inadequate in the South.
There is also a relative lack of black physicians to
help the black community acheive better health. Public
health facilities need to be established to deal with
such dreaded diseases as syphilis and tuberculosis.
Black health problems are similar to that of whites,
except in regard to the frequency of some diseases.
Only when all four areas of the situation are examined
will blacks be the beneficiaries of better health.

176. Davis, Michael M. and Smythe, Hugh H.   "Providing
Adequate Health Service to Negroes," Journal of Negro
Education 18 (1949):305-17.

Michael Davis was Chairman of the Committee on Research
in Medical Economics of the National Association for the
Advancement of Colored People (NAACP). Hugh Smythe was
Assistant Director of the Department of Special Research
for the NAACP. Notes that adequate health service

requires the availability of health personnel and
facilities, the ability of the recipients of health care
to pay for care, and the education of people in the
utilization of services and the practice of good hygiene
and nutritional habits. Points out that blacks are
disadvantaged in all three categories of requirements
dealing with adequate health care. Presents data that
indicate that black mortality rates from diseases such
as tuberculosis, syphilis, diseases of pregnancy, and
other diseases are much higher than the comparable
mortality rates for whites. Discusses three tables that
identify the inadequacy of the financial resources
available to southerners in general and to blacks in
particular with respect to paying for health care
services. Other factors hindering black health care
opportunities are the lack of personnel and facilities,
the prevalence of discrimination, and the inadequacy of
health education. Recommends three ways to alleviate
black health care problems: private charity, public
charity, and national health insurance.

177. Davis, W. A. "Some Facts Related to Negro Mortality in
the United States." Journal of the National Medical
Association 22 (1) (1930): 26-29.

The author first presents three facts regarding the
black population based on data from 1900-1910 and
1910-1920. The increase in the black population
declined by 40 percent from 1910-1920 as compared to
1900-1910. By 1920 the increase in wage earners had
declined by 15 percent despite the 6.7 percent increase
in total population. Although a healthful race normally
shows not only an increase in population but also in
wage earners, black wage earners showed an actual
decrease of 6 percent between 1910 and 1920. The author
asks why this occurred. He discounts life insurance
data since it does not apply in any way to the
uninsured. Using 1926 mortality reports of the U.S.
Bureau of the Census, he determines that the national
death rate for 1926 for all races was 12.2 with the
white rate at 10.6 while the black rate was 18.8 of 62
percent higher than that of whites. Comparison of the
race rates reveals that the black rate was 76 percent
higher than the national rate and 88 percent higher than
the white rate. His second question concerned the
section of the U.S. that has the greatest death rate and
longevity in urban and rural life. Points out that the
difference in the white urban rate of 12.7 and the rural
rate of 10.6 is 2.1 deaths per 1,000 white population as
compared with the black urban rate of 23.2 and the rural
of 15.6, a difference of 6.6 or three times greater
among blacks than among whites. Discusses the role of
tuberculosis and notes that blacks are particularly
susceptible to diseases of certain organs and systems,
especially infectious and epidemic diseases. After
summarizing his findings, the author proposes to gather
data necessary to convince the Texas legislature to
institute reforms designed to alleviate these problems.

178.   "Death and the Negro." National Negro Health News 15
(2) (April-June 1947):9.

Based on information made available by Metropolitan Life
Insurance Company, discusses the "substantially higher"
mortality rate among blacks. Specific data are given
for the 5-year period from 1942-1946. Suggests that
some leading diseases in the country take a larger toll
among blacks than whites. Among the major causes of
higher black mortality are tuberculosis, syphilis and
its sequelae, and homicide. On "The Brighter Side",
points out large declines in the mortality rate in the
preceding 35 years for a number of diseases including
pneumonia, tuberculosis, typhoid fever and the principle
communicable diseases of childhood. Discusses the
general improvement in life-expectancy among blacks as
evidence of gradual improvement in health related areas.
Concludes with praise for the "progress achieved so far"
but warns that there are many health problems among
blacks of "major proportions." Much "is yet to be done
in reducing the excessive toll of preventable disease
and premature death in this large segment of the
population."

179.   "Declining Death Rate Among Negroes," Journal of the
American Medical Association 78 (23) (June 10, 1922):1833.

A medical note, which states, "A remarkable decline has
taken place in the last decade in the mortality of
negroes," according to the Statistical Bulletin,
Metropolitan Life Insurance Company, April 22. This
company, which has more that 1,600,000 black policy
holders, reports the mortality of colored policy holders
in 1911 as 17.5 per thousand, and in 1921, 13.2 per
thousand, a decrease of 25 percent. The improvement
says the Bulletin, is not local but represents a very
broad movement affecting virtually all areas. There are
many factors acting favorably on the health of blacks,
among which is the development of health activities in
the South and Southwest. The economic status of blacks,
which has risen since the war, is also a factor favoring
black health.

180.   Deibert, Austin V.   "Cancer Among Negroes," National
Negro Health News 14 (4) (October-December 1946):5-6.

Provides a description of cancer and its treatment and
includes a list of 7 conditions which should lead one to
consult a physician for early detection purposes.
Presents a statistical summary of cancer among blacks
taken from data available for 1943. The highlights are
as follows: 1 of 16 blacks died of cancer (10,658 total;
6,387 females, 4,271 males); uterine and breast cancer
account for more than one-half of the female deaths;
stomach and prostate cancer account for most male
deaths; the age group most affected in both sexes is
50-59. Describes significant differences between the
races, sexes and localities and summarizes that: between
ages 25 and 65 cancer is more prevalent in females of

both races; uterine cancer for blacks is 63 percent
higher than for whites perhaps due to untended tears and
lacerations during childbirth; skin cancer is less
prevalent in whites than blacks because of the black
pigmentation factor; and the only significant cancer
differences between the North and South appear to be in
skin cancer figures due to greater exposure from the
sun. Among blacks, 50 percent more women die of cancer
than men. In conclusion, urges more lay-education
regarding cancer and stresses early detection as the
best remedy.

181. Deibert, Austin V. and Bruyere, Martha C. "Untreated
Syphilis in the Male Negro: III. Evidence of Cardiovascular
Abnormalities and Other Forms of Morbidity," The Journal of
Venereal Disease Information 27 (11) (November 1946):
301-314.

This study is the third in a series which examines the
progression of untreated syphilis in the black male.
Looks specifically at cardiovascular abnormalities as
well as other forms of morbidity resulting from the
untreated illness. Concludes that untreated syphilis in
the black male results in far greater physical
disability than in uninfected populations of similar
characteristics and environment and that the physical
impairment in the infected black male may be the result
of either the infection directly or increased
susceptibility to other morbidity conditions resulting
from the infection. Although the illness may not result
in immediate mortality, increased morbidity and
shortened life span are the consequences of untreated
syphilis in the black male.

182. Dent, Albert W. "Hospital Services and Facilities
Available to Negroes in the United States," Journal of Negro
Education 18 (3) (Summer 1949): 326-332.

Looks at factors that have caused black hospital access
and use to be less than that for whites. Attributes
this disparity to a number of sources including:
inadequacy of facilities, denial of the use of existing
facilities and the inability of blacks to pay for
private services. Argues that the establishment of a
Commission on Hospital Care by the American Hospital
Association and the Hill-Burton Act have done much to
improve black access to health services and the quality
of black health services. Points out that these
measures are only the beginning and much more must be
done to address the black health problem.

183. "Dental Team Serves Southern States," National Negro
Health News 18 (1950): 15.

A black dental team consisting of a dentist and two
hygienists demonstrated the use of sodium fluoride in 15
communities in Tennessee, Mississippi, Georgia, and
Alabama. The dental team applied the fluoride mixture
to more than 5,000 black children. According to the

team, the sodium fluoride when properly applied would
reduce new tooth decay by 40 percent. This
demonstration was a cooperative effort of the state
health departments and the Public Health Service.

184. Denton, William and Loveless, James A. "The Oral Use
of Sulfathiazole as a Prophylaxis for Gonorrhea," Journal of
the American Medical Association 121 (11) (March 13,
1943):827-828.

Describes an experiment to determine the effectiveness
of Sulfathiazole against gonorrhea. The drug was given
to 1400 black soldiers prior to leaving the fort on
pass. The drug proved to be effective against gonorrhea
and chanchroid as the rate dropped to a level of 8 per
thousand from 171 per thousand.

185. Deutsch, Albert. "The First United States Census of
the Insane and Its Use as Pro-Slavery Propaganda," Bulletin
of the History of Medicine 15 (1944):469-482.

Discusses the use of ethnology, the science which
investigates the mental and physical differences in man,
as a means of supporting the pro-slavery movement and
suggests studying of the shape of skulls as a means of
understanding the secrets of human reasoning. It was
therefore thought that blacks had no capacity to reason
and the skull served only as "...a sort of helmet for
resisting heavy blows." Extols the virtues of theories
that placed blacks far inferior to whites. Concludes
with census data supporting the theory of a high rate of
mental disease among southern blacks and the theory that
emancipation was to blame for the apparent rate of
increase in insanity among blacks.

186. Dickens, Dorothy and Ford, Robert N. "Geophagy (Dirt
Eating) Among Mississippi Negro School Children," American
Sociological Review 7 (February 1942): 59-65.

The authors examine the incidence of dirt eating among
school children in Oktibbeha County, Mississippi, and
why they engage in such practice. The reasons given
were that it tasted good, it was good for you, it was
good for pregnant mothers. From this, four hypotheses
are examined which attempt to explain dirt eating. A
survey was administered by the county's teachers to the
school children which asked if and how often they ate
dirt. As many as 25 percent surveyed said that they
did. A variance analysis indicated that there was a
significant relationship between dirt eating and the
number of iron-rich foods consumed. Dirt eating was
found to be more frequent among groups of people who
experienced a deficiency of iron in their diets,
especially among the black children.

187. Dill, D. B., Wilson, J. W., Hall, F. G., and Robinson,
S. "Properties of the Blood of Negroes and Whites in
Relation to Climate and Season," Journal of Biological
Chemistry 136 (1940): 449-460.

Focuses on the question of the degree of dependence of
the properties of arterial blood on weather, climate,
race, and individual makeup. Subjects consisted of
Harvard students, "colored sharecroppers" and laboratory
staff (control group). Experiment sites were Boston,
Benoit, MS, and Boulder, CO. Arterial CO_2s, aterial
pHs, and venous pHs were measured and compared between
races and climates. Though some slight differences were
observed, they generally concluded that the study failed
to produce evidence of substantial differences.

188.   "Distribution of White and Colored Physicians," Journal
of the American Medical Association 85 (26) (December 26,
1925):2051.

Per a request of a letter to the editor, a table was
published showing the number of colored and white
physicians per state as of 1924. Eleven of the 48
states had no colored physicians and seven states had
less than ten colored physicians. There was a total of
3,514 colored physicians and 143,496 white physicians.

189.   Division of Chronic Disease, Public Health Service,
FSA, "The Nutritional Status of Negroes," Journal of Negro
Education 18 (Summer 1949): 291-304.

Discusses findings obtained from surveys of black and
white families by the Nutrition Branch of the Public
Health Service. The findings show evidence of a
relatively poor nutritional condition among both races
with high levels of anemia, goiter, and skin diseases.
Some race differentials are evidenced by lower intake of
certain types of food and by higher incidence of some
physical symptoms among blacks. However, these
differentials are not consistently in one direction and
in some cases blacks demonstrate higher nutritional
status than whites.

190.   Dixon, Russell A.   "Sources of Supply of Negro Health
Personnel, Section B: Dentists," The Journal of Negro
Education 6 (1937): 477-482.

Russell cites a 1930 United States Census Report showing
the low figure of 1,773 black dentists in the entire
country. Russell notes that up to 1930 there had been a
steady increase in the training and availability of
black dentists, but due to the Depression of the early
1930's, the expectation would be for a levelling off in
the number of black dentists for the 1930-1940 period.
Notes the dire need for all races of dentists in the
South, with a 1930 figure cited of only one dentist for
every 12,312 people. The economic and social problems
of blacks in particular hinder the education and
training of a sufficient number of dentists. Points out
that stricter educational requirements had worked to the
detriment of the blacks aspiring to be dentists. Both
the educational and economic background of blacks would
have to be improved before the country could reasonably
expect to see significantly more black dentists.

191.   Doull, James A.   "Comparative Racial Immunity to
Diseases," The Journal of Negro Education 6 (1937): 429-437.

Notes the apparent and troubling susceptibility of
blacks to pulmonary tuberculosis, but also notes the
difficulty in isolating specific causes as definitive.
Doull does note, however, the clear influence the
environment has on black susceptibility to this disease.
As for the diseases of diptheria and scarlet fever, the
differences in mortality between blacks and whites
appear to lie in the greater resistance ability of the
blacks, although Doull notes that the mechanism for that
resistance could not as yet be explained. Other
diseases which cause blacks to suffer higher mortality
rates than for whites are: syphilis, gonorrhea, malaria,
tetanus, typhoid fever, and puerperal septicemia.
Observes a greater exposure rate as the cause.

192.   Downes, Jean,   "An Experiment In The Control Of
Tuberculosis Among Negroes." Milbank Memorial Fund Quarterly
28 (2) (April 1950):   127-153.

Observes that the most important tuberculosis problem is
the control of the disease among blacks. Since it was
discovered that tuberculosis mortality does vary with
the level of living of groups of the population and that
nutrition is an important environmental factor
determined to a large extent by the level of living, it
seemed important to conduct an extensive experiment to
learn whether an improved nutritional status and by
implication a higher level of living will affect the
incidence of tuberculosis among persons at risk of
attack because of exposure in the family. This
particular experiment was conducted on black families in
Harlem. A consistent effort was made throughout the
five year period of the study to meet the following
requirements to insure the validity of the experiment.
The control population had to be similar in all
essential respects to the experimental population.
Relevant data capable of evaluation and statistical
analysis had to be obtained for both populations with
equal care and exactness. The conclusions drawn from
the study have had a significant impact on the fight
against tuberculosis.

193.   "Dr. Cumming and the National Negro Health Movement."
National Negro Health News 16 (4) (1948): 18.

On March 2, 1921, Dr. Robert R. Motor, successor to Dr.
Booker T. Washington as principal of Tuskegee Institute,
addressed a letter to Surgeon General Hugh S. Cumming,
requesting the cooperation of the Public Health Service
in promoting the National Negro Health Week and in
carrying out a year-round program for the improvement of
the health of the colored population. Beginning with
the year 1921, the Public Health Service has published
each year a Health Week Bulletin, poster and school
leaflet for the use of participating state and local
health agencies and various community groups and

organizations. Also, through the services of Dr. Roscoe
C. Brown, the Public Health Service has fostered field
work in a number of states and communities.

194. Dublin, Louis I. "Recent Improvement in the Negroes'
Mortality," Opportunity 1 (4) (April 1923): 5.

A note of warning that the death rate among blacks is
too high and especially so from the diseases and
conditions which are known to be preventable. Draws
conclusions based upon the extensive experience of the
Metropolitan Life Insurance Company among blacks between
the years 1911 and 1922 which indicated that blacks have
the willingness and the capacity to increase their life
span very materially. During these years, the mortality
of the black policyholders declined from a rate of 17.5
to 13.6 per 1,000 which represents a decline of 22
percent or more than one-fifth. Notes the public health
movement among blacks is only of recent origin and the
full effect of the work would not be felt for years to
come. Provides an indication of what may be
accomplished when those states and cities which contain
many blacks increase their expenditures for public
health work, improve the sanitation of their immediate
vicinities, and take greater advantage of the knowledge
available for the prevention of disease.

195. Dublin, Louis I. "The Effect of Health Education On
Negro Mortality." Opportunity 2 (20) (August 1924):
232-234.

Presents health data concerning blacks who were insured
in the Industrial Department of the Metropolitan Life
Insurance Company. Those insured included men, women,
and children of all ages who were engaged in every
conceivable occupation. They lived almost altogether in
the towns and cities of the country. This is important
because it is especially in the cities that the health
conditions of blacks have been found very
unsatisfactory. Discusses (1) death mortality records
of the Metropolitan Life Insurance Company, (2)
tuberculosis as a cause of death among blacks, (3)
diseases which affected mostly children, (4) sanitary
conditions surrounding blacks, (5) social and
degenerative diseases, and (6) infulenza. Concludes
that blacks must learn to tinnk more and more in terms
of health as a key to improvement in other respects.

196. Dublin, Louis I. "Life, Death and the Negro," The
American Mercury 12 (September-December 1927):37-45.

This work serves as a brief history of black birth rates
and mortality rates from the seventeenth century to the
twentieth century. Census data from 1790 to 1920 are
included. Measures the percent of decennial increase in
the "colored population" for each decade and suggests
that adequate records of black health care on the slave
plantations do not exist. However, argues that black
mortality rates before the Civil War were approximately

the same as those rates for whites in southern cities
and were higher than white mortality rates in northern
cities. Black health problems came into focus during
Reconstruction. In the twentieth century, blacks
benefited from health and sanitation improvements even
though whites were the prime beneficiaries. Provides
statistics from life insurance companies that show
decreases in mortality rates for blacks for such
diseases as tuberculosis, measles, whooping cough, and
diptheria. Attributes the migration of blacks to
northern industrial cities to increases in mortality
rates from 1911 to 1926 for such diseases as
"...cerebral hemorrhage, organic diseases of the
heart,...chronic nephritis,...cancer, and diabetes."

197. Dublin, Louis I. "The Health of the Negro,"
Opportunity 6 (July 1928):198-200, 216.

Summarizes the status of black health from data
collected in 20 years of serving in the insurance
business. Recounts major improvements in the health of
the black race and observes that "a veritable revolution
in the condition of the colored race has taken place."
Asserts that blacks have indeed adjusted to their new
environment and are "capable of living advantageously in
an American environment." While noting improvement in
nearly every disease affecting blacks, emphasizes that
concentrated attention must be given to the continuing
fight against tuberculosis, syphilis and infant
mortality. In the campaign to improve black health, the
black physician is of supreme importance. For this
reason training facilities for black health care
personnel must be improved, the number of black dentists
must increased and more medical facilities must be made
available to blacks. Argues that in the treatment of
diseases among blacks, black physicians must take into
account "medical economics." As the blacks of America
are generally poor and unable to pay for adequate
medical attention, only through cooperation of agencies
willing to lower the costs of treatment can medicine and
economics be brought be brought into line. Finally,
stresses the obligation the white race must assume in
the campaign for better health among blacks for the
betterment of the health of the nation as a whole.

198. Dublin, Louis I. "The Health Of The Negro--The Outlook
For The Future." Opportunity 6 (7) (July 1928): 198-200,
216.

Provides a general overview of the health of the black
race and describes the adaptation of the black race to
the hazards of life in the United States. The black
race has proven that it is capable of living
advantageously in an American environment and that it
can profit from modern medical science to the same
degree that any other race can. Discusses the
significance of the dedication of the Howard University
Medical Building as an event of the first importance for
blacks in the history of medicine in the United States,

especially in view of the inadequate medical facilities
available for blacks. Argues that the black race is a
vigorous one with no particular weakness which make it
easy prey to disease. Blacks have no real grounds for
discouragement or for any feeling of racial inferiority.

199. Dublin, Louis I. "Health Gains Among Negroes,"
American Journal of Public Health 19 (February 1929):211-212.

A study of black Metropolitan Life Insurance Company
policyholders. Discusses differences in black and white
mortality rates. The death rate of black children age 1
to 14 improved by 38 percent in 1925-27 as compared to
1911-13. For the same category of whites, the
improvement was 43.6 percent. For the age group 15-24,
the rate of improvement for blacks and whites was 28.8
and 31.9 percent, respectively. Grim figures began to
surface for blacks over the age of 25. The improvement
for blacks was only one-half that of whites. Notes that
the single greatest reason for the improvement of the
black mortality rate for the period 1911-13 compared
with 1925-27 was the decline in the death rate from
tuberculosis. The tuberculosis death rate among blacks
insured by Metropolitan Life was 233.6 per 100,000 for
the first half of 1928. In comparison, the figure for
heart disease was 233.9 per 100,000.

200. Dublin, Louis I. "The Epidemiology of Tuberculosis of
Negroes," American Journal of Public Health 21 (March
1931):290-1.

Of the ten million black persons in the United States,
25,000 die every year from tuberculosis. The disease is
four times more fatal for blacks than whites in the
20-24 age group. The fall in death rate, more abrupt in
black women than men, is continuous throughout the
remainder of life. The total death rate, unlike that of
white people, is somewhat less in black men than in
black women. Using a pool of 2,500,000 blacks and
18,500,000 whites, the Metropolitan Life Insurance
Company study indicated that the average death rate per
100,000 from 1925-27 was 68.9 for whites and 203 for
blacks, a ratio of approximately 1 to 3. The ratio of
deaths for the two races between birth and fifteen years
of age being 1 to 9.2, age fifteen to twenty-five years
of age, 1 to 3.9. Postmortem observations suggest that
the American black escapes tuberculosis infection during
childhood more frequently that white people. In
contrast, however, blacks more often suffer in adult
life from rapidly fatal tuberculosis with the
characteristics of the first infection of white
children.

201. Dublin, Louis I. "The Health of the Negro: Striking
Progress in One Decade." Readers Digest 57 (September
1950): 50-52.

Points out that the number one criticism leveled at the
U.S. from behind the Iron Curtain concerns the manner in

which the country treats minority groups. The record of blacks in health progress provides an excellent answer to those who challenge the sincerity of our democracy. However, the over-all health status of the black population, still lags over 20 years behind the rest of the country. Much of this disparity arises from the lack of adequate black medical facilities and trained medical personnel.

202.   Dublin, Louis I., "Vital Statistics: Health Gains Among Negroes," American Journal of Public Health 19 (February 1929): 211-212.

Reports on the health gains of 2,500,000 black industrial policy holders of the Metropolitan Life Insurance Company. Argues that the death rate among insured black children ages 1 to 14 improved by 38 per cent over the past three years, 1911 to 1913,while mortality rates for whites improved by 43.6 per cent during the same period. Between ages 15 and 24 the black gain of 28.8 per cent was close to that of whites of 31.9 per cent. After age 25, black gains lessened as whites continued to improve.

203.   Dummett, Clifton O. "Improving Dentistry in the Negro Population." National Negro Health News 14 (1) (1946): 12-14.

There was a general appreciation of dentistry as one of the important phases of the over-all public health program leading to increased attention to the failings of dentistry and the importance and needs of dental care. These needs were even more acute in the case of blacks. The large majority of black dentists are graduates of the dental schools of Howard University and Meharry Medical College. In order to increase the number of black dentists more black dental schools should be opened. Another way would be to expand and improve the existing colleges. Black students should also be encouraged to apply for admission to dental schools other than Howard and Meharry. The dental profession also needs well-trained black teachers. Black dental schools must be able to compete with all other dental schools in the country.

204.   Duncan, C. Frederick. "Negro Health in Jacksonville, Florida," The Crisis 49 (January 1942): 29-32.

Explores the "regrettable health of the black in the city of Jacksonville. Black health is hampered by three factors: politics, economic conditions and ignorance. Points out that individuals armed with state authority mercilessly and consistently relegate the black into a situation of impotence. The municipality steals from him his right to go to the polls to vote. As a result there are segregated black districts and black ghettos, both characterized by poorly laid out, unpaved, sandrutted and non-lighted streets and lanes that are physical and moral hazards. Therefore, is it a wonder

that blacks are more exposed to contagious and
infectious diseases than are non-black groups.

205.   "Education of the Negro Physician," Journal of the
American Medical Association 80 (17) (April 28, 1923):1244.

An editorial which notes the concern of the country for
the protection and promotion of the health of the black
population. Observes that to best meet the health needs
of the black population, black physicians must play a
part. Notes that there are only two Class A medical
schools devoted entirely to the training of black
students. These two schools graduate about 50 a year.
Notes that many qualified applicants are turned away
because of lack of space. One problem is the lack of
funding. Suggests that the training of black physicians
is a field that might be cultivated by those who are
prepared to give financial aid to medical education.

206.   Edwards, Mary S. "Popular Health Education in Simplest
Terms: An Experience in Social Hygiene Education for Negroes
in the City of New Orleans," Journal of Social Hygiene 20 (4)
(April 1934): 177-181.

A report on a social hygiene education campaign carried
out in New Orleans. Campaign's goal was to convey to
blacks the facts concerning the dangerous communicable
disease, syphilis and gonorrhea, in order to persuade
them to avoid exposure to infection or to place
themselves under the care of a qualified physician if
already infected to protect their family and intimates
from being infected. In these public meetings, the
tools used had to be of the simplest calculated to reach
and appeal to people of low literacy. The usual printed
material and the usual media of the press and radio had
no use here, and the message of the campaign was
conveyed to its audience largely by word of mouth and
through visual means such as film showings. The health
status of blacks living in the city of New Orleans is
greatly influenced by the area's noticeable
over-crowding, gambling, flagrantly operated
prostitution, prevalent disease, poor housing and
unsanitary conditions. In 1931, statistics of venereal
disease cases under treatment in New Orleans by licensed
physicians showed twice as many black people under
treatment than whites. It was also found that the
amount of treatment administered by illegal medical
practitioners was extremely high. A survey among the
men in the city showed that at least one-half of the
white men with venereal disease and 80 percent of the
black men with venereal disease attempted either
self-treatment or were treated with drugs over the
counter before going to a doctor or clinic for
treatment. One objective of this campaign was to
educate the illiterate black to the practice of quackery
and to direct them against venereal disease.

207.   Eleazer, Robert B.   A Brief Survey of the Negro's Part in American Medical History: America's Tenth Man (Conference on Education and Race Relations, Atlanta, GA, 1933).

The census of 1920 reported 3,495 black physicians, 1,109 dentists, and 3,341 trained nurses. A number of blacks had achieved national reputation as physicians and surgeons. There were associations of black physicians and surgeons. There were associations of black physicians and dentists in nearly all the States. The leading organization was the National Medical Association. There were more than one hundred hospitals conducted by blacks. Considered as the best was the Veteran's Hospital in Tuskegee, Alabama, a $3,000,000 government enterprise which was staffed entirely by black physicians, nurses and employees. In the twelve years from 1910 to 1922 the death rate of blacks decreased thirty percent and their death rate from tuberculosis decreased fifty percent. Since 1912 the life span of blacks had increased five years.

208.   Ellis, Elaine.   "Sterilization: A Menace to the Negro," The Crisis 44 (May 1937): 137, 155.

Rather than improve the condition of the masses of the people, society is turning to sterilization. Points out that the black American would suffer most under such a law. Sterilization under a normal system, would be desirable as a strictly energetic measure. But under a social order that is motivated by competition, it is a dangerous menace to oppressed classes and races.

209.   Ellis, Elaine.   "Tuberculosis Among Negroes," Crisis 46 (4) (April 1939):112, 125.

Emphasizes that despite modern medical advances against tuberculosis, its rate among blacks still remains high, largely due to the disadvantages in economic conditions of most of the race. "Conditions placing the body at a physical disadvantage are to be found in every stratum of our population; but malnutrition, poor housing, bad working conditions, and lack of medical attention are to be found only in the lower-income groups." For example, unskilled workers have the highest incidence of tuberculosis. Similarly, blacks have higher rates of the disease than do whites who are economically better off than blacks. "The Negro population contributes 30 percent of the known cases of tuberculosis." Because conditions are even worse in the South, Southern blacks have the highest tuberculosis mortality in America. Concludes that tuberculosis among blacks can be controlled if: 1) tuberculosis is viewed as a problem of the whole population; 2) the public is educated; 3) better facilities are built in order to cope with the disease; and 4) more black doctors and nurses are trained.

210.   Embree, Edwin R.   "Negro Illness and the Nation's Health," Crisis 36 (3) (March 1929):84, 97.

Argues that black illness affects the health of the
whole nation and since diseases have no color
preference, any disease which may infect blacks may also
infect the whole population. Despite this fact, the
conditions of black health is below the conditions of
white health. Cites data in order to demonstrate the
differences between black and white mortality rates.
Between 1922 to 1925 in the state of Illinois the annual
death rate of blacks was 23 per thousand as contrasted
with 11.2 for whites. Concludes that the health of
blacks must be improved in order to improve the health
of all Americans. This may be accomplished by
"improving sanitation, good doctors and nurses who in
increasing numbers must be members of the race,
hospitals and clinics, and health education."

211. Eskridge, Louisa J. "Community-Wide Cooperation for
Better Health and Sanitation," National Negro Health News 14
(4) (October-December 1946): 1-4.

Seeks to answer the following question: "What guiding
principles can be applied to the problem of cooperation
in public health as one of many community needs?" One
partial answer is indicated in "hundreds" of current
community projects in which citizens participate
primarily because of focus on the specific problem
rather that the difficulties of communal cooperation
(i.e. race, religion, economic status). The projects
cited include leadership training workshops for public
health, mother-daughter groups for improved maternal and
infant health, public health education, mass x-ray
surveys, and Southwest Indians meeting with government
officials to determine health needs among their people.
The conclusion outlines steps for the professional
worker or individual citizen to follow for successful
communal cooperation for improvement in health and
sanitation. These steps are: 1) recognize that
communal activity is already going on; 2) join existing
groups; 3) use existing resources; 4) start with people
who work together; 5) identify the problem with them; 6)
use interested people; 7) use emerging community
leaders; and 8) begin in the community.

212. Evans, L. S. "Addison's Disease: Three Cases,"
American Journal of Medical Science 176 (October
1928):499-503.

Addison's disease, a relatively rare disorder with
interesting racial implications, formed the subject of a
number of racially-defined medical studies in the early
years of this century. This disease is characterized by
extreme weakness in the victims, who also suffer from
low blood pressure and a brownish discoloration of the
skin due to the decreased secretion of cortisol from the
adrenal cortex, which is the cause of hypoadrenalism.

213. Ewing, Oscar R. "The President's Health Program and
the Negro," Journal of Negro Education 18 (1949):436-43.

The author, Federal Security Administrator, describes
the national health care bill proposed by President
Harry Truman. Notes that blacks have suffered from
maldistribution of health personnel and facilities and
the high costs of medical care. The answer to the
problem for blacks is the same answer for the 50 percent
of Americans who can afford more than minimal health
care: nationalized health care. The social insurance
program of the President was to be extended to everyone
except rural farm workers by deducting 1½ percent of
payroll income of workers and requiring employers to
match the 1½ percent. Farm and domestic workers would
be aided by future legislation. The infirmed and
unemployed would be covered because of the fact that
local public and private agencies would pay the
premiums. Also important was the inclusion of the
guarantee that "no discrimination as to race, creed, and
color" was allowed by the plan. In addition to social
health insurance, the author promised more federal aid
for the building of hospitals and the training of black
and white medical personnel. Finally, recognizes that
national health insurance was a part of the President's
longer struggle for the civil rights of black Americans.

214. Farmer, Harold E. "An Account of the Earliest Colored
Gentlemen in Medical Science in the United States," Bulletin
of the History of Medicine 8 (1940):599-618.

A paper presented before the College of Physicians of
Philadelphia in 1939 which discusses the many black
"doctors" of the early slave periods and the various
forms of medicine that they practiced, such as
blood-letting. Also discusses other educated and
trained black physicians throughout history including
black dentists and the existence and contributions of
black medical societies.

215. Fetter, Ferdinand and Howell, John C. "Sickle Cell
Anemia and Carcinoma of the Breast Complicated by Pregnancy,"
Annals of Internal Medicine 32 (January-June 1950):548-553.

Presents the case of a 28 year old black woman who is
pregnant, has sickle cell anemia and carcinoma of the
breast. A macerated fetus was born four days after
radical mastectomy. The patient died nine and one-half
months after mastectomy from metastases. Sickle cell
anemia was considered a factor in her death. The
unfavorable effects of pregnancy on sickle cell anemia
and carcinoma of the breast are discussed.

216. Fitts, John B. "Syphilis of the Stomach - A Study of
Eight Cases," Annals of Internal Medicine 4 (1930/31):
628-631.

The case studies of eight black males are reviewed and
reference is made to the actual involvement of the
stomach in the syphilitic process, so-called gastric
syphilis. The material used is derived from the medical
wards of a hospital where the admission of the Southern

black is utilized for teaching purposes. In conclusion, the following is offered: (1) there were only eight cases of gastric syphilis in 35,000 admissions; (2) comment is made on the occurrence of so few cases in such a large syphilitic material; (3) pain, vomiting, loss of weight, positive blood Wassermann and characteristic x-ray findings are symptoms in gastric syphilis; (4) one should avoid attributing all gastric symptoms to an existing constitutional syphilis, as they may be entirely independent of each other; and (5) syphilis may be the etiologic factor in the investigation of chronic disease of the gastro-intentional tract.

217.   Forbes, W. H., Johnson, R. E. and Consolazio, F. "Leukopenia in Negro Workmen," The American Journal of Medical Sciences 201 (3) (March 1941): 407-412.

This study resulted from earlier research on the physiology of black sharecroppers in Mississippi which had indicated a large incidence of leukopenia. The researchers found leukopenia and slightly lower erythrocyte levels and oxygen capacities among black sharecroppers in Mississippi than for whites in the area. This leukopenia was principally neutropenia, but involved the lymphocytes as well in some cases. Administration of iron resulted in a marked increase in the leukocyte count in ten of the twelve selected sharecroppers. Curiously, white sharecroppers in the same region eating similar diets showed no leukopenia. The researchers suggest the possibility that the leukopenia found in the black sharecroppers in Mississippi may be a local racial characteristic worthy of record.

218.   Foster, Robert H.   "Paresis in the Negro," American Journal of Psychiatry 82 (April 1926): 630-638.

Discusses the misconception that paresis is not frequently found in cases in syphilis and argues that paresis is more common in the Southern black than in the Southern white. According to the data presented from seven large North American hospitals, whites had a paresis of 11.2 percent for males and 3 percent for females while blacks had a rate of 28 percent and 11 percent, respectfully. Observes that 40 years ago the incidence of paresis was rare; but with the increase of disease among blacks, paresis as a condition is spreading. Concludes that: paresis is more frequent in the black than the white race; the neurological changes are well marked; there is a difference in the mental picture caused by the environment and racial characteristics; and the remissions are less often found, but that the course is more rapid than in the white race.

219.   Fox, Edna P.   "Social Health Conditions Among Virginia Negroes," Southern Workman 53 (August 1924): 371-373.

The author notes that better health conditions enable
the black people of Virginia to take more advantages of
educational opportunities, since ignorance is related to
the spread of disease. Blacks take pride in having
clean schoolrooms which reflects pride in themselves and
black school children are neat because they are taught
simple health rules. The State Bureau of Social Hygiene
aids churches and other organizations that stress the
importance of good health. However, the State Health
Board has been crippled by cutbacks in funding by the
legislature. To compensate for this, black colleges are
urged to implement social hygiene courses. The author
concludes that there should be more education not only
on social hygiene but on venereal disease and its
effects.

220. Frazier, Chester N.   "The Problem of Syphilis in the
Negro Race", Texas State Reports on Biology and Medicine 6
(2) (Summer 1948): 192-199.

A discussion of the variance of syphilis cases in Texas
and other states. Initially, the author remarks that,
"In considering the racial implications of syphilis it
is not the individual Negroes or the individual white
man who concerns us most. It is the community of
Negroes or Caucasians, who comprise a geographical unit,
that determines the force of morbidity which syphilis
exerts on race." Concludes with data that indicate
variance in contraction of the disease. "Among Negro
males between 21 and 35 years of age, the rate in Texas
was 343.3 per 1,000, and among white males it was 53.4
per 1,000." "In Rhode Island the Negro rate was 91.8
per 1,000 against 343.3 per 1,000 in Texas. In
Wisconsin where the white race fared best, the rate was
6.4 per 1,000 in contrast to 53.4 per 1,000 whites in
Texas." Thus, the problem of syphilis is more
pronounced in Texan blacks than in whites; however, both
blacks and whites have a higher rate of incidence of
syphilis in Texas than in other states.

221. Gardner, George E. and Aaron, Sadie.   "The Childhood
and Adolescent Adjustment of Negro Psychiatric Casualties,"
American Journal of Orthopsychiatry 16 (3) (July
1946):481-495.

A study of the social, cultural, and economic
backgrounds of black naval men who have been admitted to
the psychiatric wards of naval hospitals. These men are
classified as "psychiatric casualties." Examines "the
possible differences in the early adjustments of the
black patient with those of the non-patient black group.
The authors are interested in "whatever differences of
similarities which might exist in the childhood and
adolescent experiences of blacks who failed to adjust to
such degree in the naval service that they were
transferred to a naval hospital for observation as to
sanity and competence." Not only were these men
compared to "normal" blacks, they were also compared to
whites who had been admitted to the psychiatric wards

because they had failed to adjust in the Navy. The
white patients and the "normal" black group were
considered the control groups. Concludes that
constitutional, familial development, social, and
economic factors found in their previous studies of
maladjustment during childhood and adjustment of
children and adolescents years in the white population
were found to exist (in some instances to an even
greater degree) among the maladjusted members of the
black race. Observes that further studies are necessary
in order to understand or explain black behavior.

222. Garrett, H. E. "Comparison of Negro and White Recruits
on the Army Tests Given in 1917-1918," The American Journal
of Psychology 58 (1945): 480-495.

The author challenges the conclusions of M. F. Montagu
(author of Intelligence of Northern Negroes and Southern
Whites in the First World War). Points out certain
errors in interpretation of the Beta and Alpha scores
obtained in the earlier study and asserts that the
method of comparison of scores was misleading.
Maintains that Alpha and Beta medians are of little
psychological value. Includes several tables giving
Alpha and Beta scores along various parameters (i.e.,
white draftees, black draftees, Northern versus Southern
blacks, etc.).

223. Garvin, Charles H. "Negro Health," Opportunity 2 (23)
(November 1924): 341-342.

Explains that any proper program of health must contain
two inter-dependent functions, one educational and the
other medical. The purpose of the first is to transfer
into conduct the principles of healthful living, and the
second is to remove the obstacles in the way of
healthful living. In New York City, two persons out of
every 1,000 died 50 years ago, but in 1920 only one died
- a total saving of 116,285 lives annually. This is a
result of improved health programs for all persons.
Emphasizes the view that blacks have been so occupied in
the struggle for existence that until now the question
of black health studied from a preventive standpoint had
been left to others. Points out that the establishment
of the School of Hygiene at Howard University School of
Medicine in Washington, D.C. marked the first major move
to have the black physician and worker take a part in
this work. Suggests that a comprehensive health program
depends upon the realization that the black race is not
a more isolated group.

224. Garvin, Charles H. "Immunity to Disease Among
Dark-Skinned People," Opportunity 4 (August 1926): 242-245.

A description of various types of
immunity-acquired-natural, racial, and individual.
Points out that immunity to certain diseases takes time
to develop into a racial immunity and cites examples
from the Senegalese, Sudanese, Egyptians and Chinese in

regard to their incidences of tuberculosis, a disease
which is known to be "no respecter of races." Concludes
that diseases are more virulent when first introduced to
a people, that blacks are more susceptible to
tuberculosis because their resistance has not had time
to build up and that "there is no doubt that the
dark-skinned races are prone to fibro-plastic processes
(fibroma)."

225.   Garvin, Charles H.   "White Plague and Black Folk,"
Opportunity 8 (8) (August 1930): 232-235.

Observes that tuberculosis is ubiquitous. It is no
respecter of race or creed and attacks irrespective of
social or economic status. Notes that thirty years ago
Dr. Frederick Hoffman in his book, Race Traits and
Tendencies of the American Negro, the following
pseudo-scientific statement was made, "The colored race
is bound to be on the downward grade...when disease will
be more destructive, vital resistance still lower, when
the number of births will fall below the deaths and
gradual extinction of the race will take place." Time
has proven this "Prophet of Negro Extinction" to be in
error. Dr. Hoffman failed to consider the fundamental
question of racial immunity to disease. Points out that
there is a difference in susceptibility or resistance to
disease that has been acquired through the years by
races of people and especially by blacks to
tuberculosis. This susceptibility has an influence on
the struggle for life and the upward or downward course
of a race.

226.   Gates, R. Ruggles.   "Pedigrees of Negro Families,"
American Journal of Psychiatry 107 (June/July 1950-51):
393-396.

Adds new literature toward the time when pedigrees from
all races can be numerous enough for statistical
evaluation of inheritance patterns. Discusses myopia,
strabismus, deafmutism, lack of sweat-glands, and
epilepsy along with normal traits and the biological
factors along with the social challenges of blacks.
Concludes that together, these two factors contribute to
the incidence of such cases in blacks as compared to
whites.

227.   Gebhart, John C.   "Syphilis as a Prenatal Problem,"
Journal of Social Hygiene 10 (4) (August 1924): 208-217.

Discusses syphilis as a complicating factor in maternal
and infant health. Dr. Haven Everson, while
Commissioner of Health for New York City, became
concerned over the high infant and maternal mortality
prevailing in the colored district, west and north of
Columbus, known as Columbus Hill. Improving the
condition of the poor began with an intensive
educational nursing service for expectant mothers in
that area in April 1917. During the following six
years, 1224 births occurred. More than half of the

mothers received at least three months prenatal care.
The puerperal death rate per 1000 deliveries for mothers
who had less than three months' care was 10.6 and 4.6
per 1000 for those who had had three months' care. The
death rate per 1000 births within the first month was
49.8 for mothers with less than three months' care and
20.6 for mothers with at least three months' care.
Where the length of prenatal care was adequate, the
mortality rate for mothers and babies was reduced by
more than 50 percent. When the rates for this district
were compared with the prevailing rates among blacks in
a similar district (Harlem or Manhattan borough), it is
obvious that there has been a saving of lives as a
result of the combined prenatal nursing and hospital
service. These findings lend to the growing conviction
that prenatal care will secure optimum results when
provisions are made for syphilitic treatment and nursing
follow-up. It is generally recognized by medical
physicians that syphilis is one of the leading causes of
miscarriages and still births. Presents a striking
picture of the toll which syphilis exacts on early
infant life by using tables summarizing clinical
findings. Contends that the findings serve as a
concrete example of the type of prenatal services needed
for the health and protection of black mothers and
babies.

228.   "A Generation Behind." Time 49 (April 7, 1947):   58.

Black health still lag a full generation behind that of
U.S. whites. Point outs some important facts about the
life expectancy of Blacks. The death rate of blacks is
33 percent higher than that of whites. Most of the
major killers that are more prevalent among blacks are
tuberculosis, kidney disease, and pneumonia. Blacks
have only 124 hospitals of their own.

229.   Gerwig, Walter H., Jr.   "Diagnosis and Treatment of
Cystosarcoma Phyllodes," Postgraduate Medicine 5 (March
1949): 219-223.

A case report of a tumor, removed from a 40 year old
black woman. The tumor weighed 17.2 pounds, was
histologically benign, and had been present 11 years,
enlarging rapidly during the last 2 years. A simple
mastectomy was performed and no recurrence occurred in
the following 4 years.

230.   Gesell, Arnold.   "Clinical Mongolism in Colored Races,"
Journal of the American Medical Association 106 (14) (May 6,
1935):1146-1150.

A discussion of mongolism among blacks. After a letter
writing campaign to various institutions for the
"feeble-minded", it was discovered that the incidence of
black mongolism was low but more frequent than commonly
supposed.

78   Annotated Bibliography

231. Glotzer, S. "Myocardial Infarction in the Negro", New York State Journal of Medicine 59 (3) (July 15, 1959): 2721.

Begins with the observation, "Although evidence indicates a positive effect of high intake of saturated fat on coronary arteriosclerosis, it is felt in the American Negro there is some doubt. [Yet], "A remarkably low incidence of myocardial infarction among low income Negroes has been found at King's County Hospital in New York City." Discusses anatomical differences in Bantu and black hearts which may be the reason for the low incidence of myocardial infarction. Concludes that further study of the black heart anatomy is needed.

232. Granger, Lester B. "The Negro Physician and Socialized Medicine," Opportunity 11 (12) (December 1933): 370-371.

Discusses the controversy surrounding the costs of medical care and its racial implications toward the black medical practitioner. Indifference occurs over the recommendations made that the costs of medical care to the average American family be reduced and that its service be made more widely available through state control or group insurance. On one side, many notable figures in the medical profession, backed by the leaders of social thought, maintain that present costs of medical attention are too high for the average family, while the service is seriously inadequate for those families and groups most in need of it. On the other side are those physicians who maintain with honest sincerity that increased socialization of medicine in the direction recommended would be a grave mistake, certain to lower the standards of the medical profession. They feel that the personal relationship between the average physician and his patients should not be removed because medicine, they insist, is a highly individualized profession. Suggests that in this situation, the black physician appears to be where the impact is hardest and the margin of protection thinnest.

233. Granger, William R.R. "A Neglected Health Problem," Opportunity 6 (March 1928): 72-73.

The "neglected health problem" which is addressed is syphilis (along with its sequelae). Citing data on incidences of syphilis in black men, women and children, contends that syphilis alone is responsible for the higher death rate among blacks. Points out that syphilis is more prevalent among blacks than whites. Concludes that "Syphilis is increasing and its hold is strongest on the Negro race."

234. Grant, Faye and Groom, Gale. "A Dietary Study Among a Group of Southern Negroes", Journal of the American Dietetic Association 35 (3) (September 1959): 910-918.

A dietary study in the Charleston, South Carolina area which points out several observations about the health

and nutrition of blacks. First, it appears that very
few blacks that were studied were actually malnourished
from a caloric view. The question, however, was not
whether the caloric intake was enough, but whether the
value of those calories taken was sufficient to maintain
good health. Everyone except the very lowest income
group obtained the required amount of the necessary
amino acids. These figures were compared to a
complementary study that was done in Haiti. It appears
that in the United States, the enriched foods, (wheat,
corn meal, etc.) which are relatively cheap, make a
definite impact on the health of blacks. The study done
in Haiti (where the grains are not enriched), shows even
higher percentages of blacks not getting the proper
amino acids, which of course, are essential to a healthy
life. Concludes that while there are some definite
problems with the health of the very lowest income
Southern blacks, the situation could be much worse
without our country's enrichments of grains with various
nutrients.

235. Graves, M. L. "Practical Remedial Measures For The
Improvement of Hygienic Conditions of The Negroes In The
South," American Journal of Public Health 16 (August 1926):
213-217.

Discusses census figures of 1910 which suggests that
miscegenation and adultery is actually increasing.
Illnesses and death among blacks account for an economic
loss of $300,000,000 yearly to the South. Suggests that
the health problem should be one of a national concern
with a private philantrophy among southern whites to
finance a Commission of Research to investigate and
improve health conditions in the South in collaboration
with black education institutions, public schools,
churches, landlords, social welfare workers, and state,
county and municipal health departments.

236. Greene, J. E. "Analyses of Racial Differences Within
Seven Clinical Categories of White and Negro Mental Patients
in the Georgia State Hospital, 1932-34," Journal of Social
Forces 17 (December 1938): 201-211.

Makes comparisons between black and white mental
patients in Georgia based on seven selected disorder
categories: senile psychoses, psychoses with cerebral
arteriosclerosis, general paralysis, psychoses with
cerebral syphilis, dementia praecox psychoses, and other
mental disorders of every type. Each sex separately is
compared to standard rates, median differences, and
percentage differences. Concludes that Georgia black
mental patients have a generally unfavorable status
compared with white patients and that Georgia blacks are
hospitalized at earlier ages, die during shorter periods
of hospital residence, and die at much earlier ages than
do Georgia whites. However, Georgia blacks have higher
percentages of discharge statuses classified as
"recovered" and "improved" than do whites.

237. Grover, Mary. "Trend of Mortality Among Southern
Negroes Since 1920," Journal of Negro Education 6
(1937):276-88.

A study of data compiled by an Associate Statistician
for the U.S. Public Health Service. The concentration
is on Southern states from 1920-1933. Data from
Arkansas, Alabama, Georgia, and Texas were excluded from
the study because of the inaccuracy of the records. The
data reveal that black death rates declined for blacks
younger than age thirty (based on "age at year 1930")
but rose for black older than age twenty-nine between
early 1920s and 1930s. Death rates for whites in the
same time period rose only in age groups above age
forty-four. In every age cohort, black death rates
exceed white death rates. In addition, white rates
dropped more than black rates over the period studied.
Black infant mortality was also higher than white infant
mortality. Certain diseases caused greater loss of life
in the black community in the 1930s relative to the
1920s. Syphilis, pellagra, and cerebral hemorrhage
deaths rose in the black community at the same time they
were falling in the white community. Deaths from
cancer, heart disease, diseases of the arteries, and
kidney diseases were up for both racial groups. Death
rates from tuberculosis, cancer, heart disease, and
cardiovascular renal diseases became more acute for
blacks in relation to whites from the period 1921-1933.
Thus, while blacks undeniably have benefited from
medical science discoveries (particularly in the area of
childhood diseases), they have not benefited as much as
whites.

238. Grover, Mary. "Negro Mortality: Mortality From All
Causes in the Death Registration States," Public Health
Reports 61 (8) (February 22, 1946):259-265.

A compilation of black mortality from all causes.
Observes that both black and white mortality had
declined from 1940 to 1946 with the black mortality
rates being higher. The black mortality rate of
decline, however was more rapid than that of whites.
The most rapid rate of decline was in the 1-4 year age
group (for both whites and blacks). As a whole, the
rate of decline of black mortality was very encouraging
especially for those under 25 years of age.

239. Grover, Mary. "Negro Mortality: The Birth Rate and
Infant and Maternal Mortality," Public Health Reports 61 (43)
(October 25, 1946):1529-1538.

Addresses the issue of black infant natality and
mortality during the 1920's to 1940's. From 1930 to
1934 there was an unusually high birth rate among blacks
and then from 1940 to 1943, natality increased 2.5
percent. Infant mortality, however was approximately 65
percent higher for blacks than for whites. Concludes
that from 1920 to 1936 natality, infant mortality, and
maternal mortality were declining at approximately the

same rate. In addition, maternal mortality is higher
among blacks than whites and higher in the South than in
the North.

240. Grover, Mary. "Negro Mortality," Public Health Reports
63 (7) (February 3, 1948):201-213.

Uses data available from the United States Bureau of
Census for a discussion detailing black mortality from
specific causes. Diseases such as diptheria, scarlet
fever, and whopping cough were charted showing death
rates for various years for whites and non-whites.
Communicable diseases in whites showed rapid decreases
during the years studied. The slower decrease in
non-whites was because of a lower rate of immunization
and less extensive use of sulfa-compounds.

241. Grover, Mary. "Physical Impairments of Members of
Low-Income Farm Families," Public Health Reports 63 (August
20, 1948): 1083-1101.

A study in 1940 of 2,447 farm owner families receiving
rehabilitation loans from the Farm Security
Administration. The findings revealed that the
age-specific mean systolic blood pressures of both males
and females were definitely above those recorded for
other groups, mainly urban. Blood pressure findings for
black farm families exhibited the same general
characteristics as those for the white families; mean
systolic and diastolic pressures were higher for blacks
in specific age groups, particularly for black women
aged 35-54; mean diastolic blood pressure for the farm
group, however, did not show much difference from that
recorded for urban groups.

242. Grover, Mary. "The Physical Defects of White and Negro
Families Examined by the Farm Security Administration, 1940,"
The Journal of Negro Education 18 (Summer 1949): 251-264.

The Farm Security Administration (FHA) conducted
physical examinations of farm families as part of the
rural borrower rehabilitation program. The purpose was
to determine the health status of rural populations in
communities where borrowing was in effect in order to
establish permanent health centers. FHA made the
following findings on the prevalence of special defects:
(1) blacks had less dental caries, less incidence of
defective vision and hearing, less diseased tonsils and
less deviated septum than whites; (2) mean blood
pressure, the percentage of high blood pressure, the
incidence of hypertension and diagnosed heart disease
were higher for blacks than for whites; (3) and black
children had been immunized less often (30 percent) than
white children.

243. Grover, Victor. "The Clinical Manifestations of Sickle
Cell Anemia," Annals of Internal Medicine 26 (1947): 843-851.

In 1910, J. B. Herrick first reported the association of sickle shaped erythrocytes with severe anemia and certain clinical symptoms now recognized as sickle cell anemia. From January, 1936 to January, 1946 there were 48 cases of active sickle cell anemia treated at Kings County Hospital. These were the clinical manifestations tabulated for this study. All patients data with only the trait (sicklemia) were used. All of the patients were black. Their ages ranged from under 4 years to 39 years. Areas of concentration noted were: duration of symptoms, sex (24 males and 24 females), sibling (7 cases of brother and sister), temperature, pulse, blood pressure, chief complaint and associated prominent symptoms or signs, ulcers of the legs, roetgenograms of the bones, skulls, and heart, electrocardiograms, blood counts, reticulocyte counts, icteric index and deaths. The previous concept of the clinical features of this disease are confirmed, but particular attention is directed to the frequent occurence of the following manifestations: (1) cardiac enlargement, (2) the presence of diastolic as well as systolic murmurs of the heart, (3) prologation of the P-R interval, (4) roentgenographic changes in the osseous system, (5) rapid and marked changes in the size of the liver and spleen, (6) neuropsychiatric signs and symptoms especially mental deficiency, and (7) abdominal crises. Two unusual manifestations were the demonstration of esphogram of auricular enlargement in two cases, and the relief of pripism by roetgen therapy.

244. Hamilton, J. F. "A Case of Sickle Cell Anemia," United States Veterans' Bureau Medical Bulletin 2 (5) (May 1926): 497-500.

Notes the case of a 33 year old black farmer admitted to a Veterans Administration (VA) Hospital. In 1918, the patient suffered his first severe attack of pain in his limbs while on a train trip. Later limb pains were felt during army drill exercises. In 1922, the patient suffered from gall stones and varicose veins. In 1925, the patient entered the VA hospital with pain in his limbs, joints, and gall bladder, as well as with a subnormal temperature. Blood tests were subsequently administered. Terms this patient "a classic case" and concludes that "the more or less apparent simultaneous rise and fall in the total number of red and white corpuscles in the blood of this patient allows one to suspect an influence, the kind and nature of which is unknown, which operates in destroying or impeding production, or both, of the two blood elements."

245. Harding, Henry O. "Health Opportunities in Harlem," Opportunity 4 (December 1926): 386-387.

Describes the services of the Harlem Committee of the New York Tuberculosis and Health Association which was organized in August, 1922. This Committee provides an Information Service for physicians treating tuberculosis patients and to individuals needing advice on health

problems. Among its services to the community are the
distribution of health-related pamphlets, a daily dental
clinic which treats up to 24 children a day using
volunteer dentists. The children who come to this
clinic are weighed and measured and assistance, advice
is given to parents whose children exhibit deficiences,
and weekly nutrition and health club meetings are held
for children in an effort to promote general good
health. In order to be of assistance to physicians, an
institute was initiated in 1923. Community health
lectures are arranged by the Committee which also loans
out posters and pamphlets to schools and other community
organizations. Funding for the Committee is provided by
the New York Tuberculosis and Health Association.

246. Harris, H.L. "Health of the Negro Family in Chicago,
Ill.," Opportunity 5 (September 1927): 258-260.

Discusses the Olivet Kindergarten Classes and Health
Work begun as a nutrition class by the Elizabeth
McCormick Memorial Fund. A program of careful
measurement and evaluation of children participating in
the 'general health and nutrition' school showed most
with normal growth and development. In comparison with
other similar but "out-patient" classes, the children at
Olivet showed few evidences of rachitic deformity which
led the author to observe that "The difference in
economic and cultural opportunities between the two
groups is, of course, the obvious answer." Concludes
that the ultimate solution to improved health in black
families lies in the coordination of all pertinent
groups in the community "to bring to every child in
every community all the forces which make possible a
satisfactory physical, mental, moral, and social
development."

247. Harris, H. L. "Negro Mortality Rates in Chicago,"
Social Service Review 1 (1) (March 1927): 58-77.

Comparative mortality rates compiled by the Chicago
Department of Health show wide discrepancies in the
rates between the white and black populations for
certain diseases. The black rates for diseases such as
tuberculosis, heart disease, and pneumonia, in which
care and sanitation play a very important part, are much
higher than the rates for the whites. The black death
rate in Chicago is more than twice that of the city's
white population. Notes that environmental factors
possibly contribute to this aspect. The insanitary
housing conditions and public health care for blacks is
poor. Suggests that efforts of black and white leaders
must be combined under a common leadership. The problem
needs to be recognized as a municipal rather than a
black problem.

248. Hartnett, W. G. "Study in Hypertension on Southern
Negroes," Southern Medical Journal 41 (September 1948):
847-848.

Examines hypertension in the Southern black because of
the diversified opinions about the occurence. Reviews
seven thousand admissions to the Mississippi Veterans
Hospital. Thirty-five percent were black. Observes
that the incidence of blacks with hypertension was
slightly higher than those patients in the white race.
Concludes that plantation blacks are not less subject to
hypertension than his northern city brother and that
military service might have contributed, to psychic
trauma as a potential cause of veterans hypertension in
evaluating the difference between the plantation and the
urban black.

249. Harvey, B. C. H. "Problems of the Colored Student,"
Journal of Medical Education 4 (1929):208-210.

A brief discussion of the problems of black students in
northern schools. Commends the 'superior colored
student' who is able to work outside of going to school.
Makes special note that the colored student needs help
in his clinical years. That is, help in getting
clerkships and other work in hospitals without color
being an issue. Finally, observes that one of the best
ways to help the colored student is to send them to
Meharry or Howard, and to look to the future of
developing other medical schools.

250. Harvey, Jane E. B. "When Children Talk Health,"
Opportunity 3 (36) (December 1925).

Begins with an excerpt from one of the essays presented
by a fourth grade black child for a composition
conducted in a school emphasizing child health work.
The health campaign is led by Mrs. Madeline Tillman, a
member of the nutrition staff of the Philadelphia
Inter-State Dairy Council. Activities consist of a
number of health stories and plays in which the children
are not only interested listeners but active
participants. Through the children, the mothers became
interested in the health rules being taught. Believes
that this teaching forms a valuable link between home
and school in bringing knowledge of the need for better
health to the whole community. The work of the Dairy
Council, through Mrs. Tillman, carries on various
activities over a radius of 150 to 250 miles with
Philadelphia as a central point. This kind of work
commands the attention of educators and has an influence
on the conduct of health instruction for the future.

251. Haynes, Elizabeth. "The Health of Negro Domestic
Workers," Journal of Negro History 4 (October 1923): 432.

Questions why agencies employing domestic workers do not
keep records relative to the worker's health. Contends
that record keeping is important because of the nature
of their work, the homes into which they go and because
their support depends on their physical ability to work.
In 1899, 80 percent of 153 male workers and 74 percent
of 395 female domestic workers in Philadelphia had been

ill during the year. Consumption, lagrippe, quinsy, sore throat, rheumatism, neuralgia, fever, dyspepsia, and chills were the most prevalent disabilities among them. There is a high incidence of infection due to the ill health of domestic workers. In 1922, women domestic workers reporting at the United States Employment Agency, Washington, D.C. said that their most common complaints were lagrippe, surgical operations, heart trouble, indigestion, neuralgia and weak back. There were five evident cases of mental disturbances. Three cases of tuberculosis were reported. The Agency indicated that such persons were not used in the home about food, yet they were employed as household maids.

252. Hazen, H. H. "A Leading Cause of Death Among Negroes: Syphilis," Journal of Negro Education 6 (1937):310-21.

The author, Professor of Dermatology and Syphilology at the Howard University School of Medicine, is concerned with the detection and treatment of syphilis in American blacks. Describes nine methods of estimating the number of incidences of syphilis and provides data that indicate that blacks are more likely than whites to suffer from syphilis and more likely to go untreated until the late stages of the disease. Other data illustrate that black women suffer much higher rates than white women (and at earlier ages), incidences of congenital syphilis in blacks are as high as 16 percent, 19 percent in some cities, and mortality rates for blacks increase (particularly for black males) at the same time white mortality rates for syphilis decrease (1912-1929). Points out that incidences of syphilis cause economic hardship for society and for the individuals by disabling black workers, causing industrial accidents (the result of neuro syphilis), causing someone to pay for treatment and causing facilities for the treatment of the victims to be built. Recommends financial commitments from society to train black doctors and to increase facilities in the present so that long-term costs associated with mounting infection rates can be alleviated.

253. Hazen, H. H., Howard, William J., Freeman, C. Wendell, and Scull, Ralph H. "The Treatment of Granuloma Inguinale in the Negro," Journal of the American Medical Association 99 (17) (October 22, 1932):1410-1411.

Reviews the history of the treatment of granuloma inguinale, various articles discussing the disease, the few cases found in white individuals and concludes that the disease was a common occurrence among blacks in Washington, D.C.. Finds that effective results are obtained by a freshly prepared solution of antimony and potassium tartrate or injections of ampules of antimony thioglycollamide.

254. Heine, Ralph W. "The Negro Patient in Psychotherapy," Journal of Clinical Psychology 6 (3) (July 1950): 373-376.

Presents some factors as to how the black population has literally been isolated from obtaining psychotherapy. "As a racial minority which has been low on the socio-economic scale, most private sources of psychotherapeutic help have been virtually closed to all but a very few Negroes." Points out that many of the emotional responses of the black patients are due to the fact they are part of a system which holds a double standard towards blacks. Thus, an understanding of why certain character reactions and emotional instabilities occur in the black community is initiated. Therefore, a firmer grip on the scope of emotional care for blacks is illicited.

255. Heller, J. R. and Bruyere, P. T. "Untreated Syphilis in the Negro Male: II. Mortality During 12 Years of Observation," The Journal of Venereal Disease Information 27 (2) (February 1946): 34-38.

This study is the second in a series which examines untreated syphilis in the black male. The focus is to determine the effect of the syphilis infection on the life span of the human host. The study group consisted of 410 black men with untreated syphilis and a comparable group of 201 uninfected black men. The study determined that untreated syphilis does reduce the life span of its host. Concludes by noting that black men between the ages of 25 and 50 with untreated syphilis can expect to have their life span reduced by 20 percent.

256. Henderson, Rose. "Health Gains for Negroes," Southern Workman 62 (August 1933): 336-341.

Notes evidence in improvements of the health of colored people in the United States. The number of tuberculosis deaths has fallen. Obviously, the low economic status of blacks and prejudice against their race have contributed to inferior health conditions. The author observes that education, extension of health and medical services via social service centers, and improvements of health work through colored doctors, nurses and racial leaders have lead to improvements. Discusses various organizations and their efforts in communities (i.e. Bureau of Crime Prevention, Children's Bureau) and increased opportunities for black interns.

257. Henegan, L. Herbert. "Keeping Well Babies Well," Crisis 41 (10) (October 1934):297, 306.

A discussion of how Kansas City, Missouri has reduced its black infant mortality rate 100 percent. "For three successive years, Kansas City, Missouri, has been rated first in the annual Negro Health Week campaigns." The success of the program is attributed to Kansas City's year-round program to combat health problems. In 1922 the city opened its first "Colored Child Welfare Station" admitted only healthy babies on Thursday mornings. Cases of illness were referred to the

municipal hospital. The purpose of the clinic was to
make sure that the healthy babies remained healthy. The
staff of the clinic knew this could only be accomplished
by encouraging mothers to bring their children to the
clinic for regular visits. Two other stations were
later opened. As a result of the clinics, black infant
mortality has decreased by almost 100 percent since
1925. After 1925 Kansas City became an important
medical center for blacks. Kansas City's commitment to
health care is "the result of long-range planning,
diligence and sacrifice on the part of citizens, both
professional and laymen, white, and colored."

258. Hesbacher, Edwin N. "A Study of Syphilis in a Negro
High School in the City of Baltimore, 1939-1943," The Journal
of Venereal Disease Information 27 (8) (August 1946):
200-204.

Reports two serologic surveys of black high school
students in Baltimore. Finds that approximately three
percent of the high school students are infected with
the disease with fifty percent of these students testing
positive for the disease under the age of fifteen. A
three year follow-up study of three quarters of the
students who had tested negative for the disease took
place next. The final results indicated that 6.3
percent of all individuals tested were found to have the
disease. The researchers found females to be infected
earlier in life than males. The infection rate was also
higher for females in the tested group, 7.4 percent for
females compared to 4.3 percent for males.

259. Heyman, Albert and Beeson, Paul B. "Studies on
Chancroid. III. Ducrey Skin Reactions in Negro Hospital
Patients," The Journal of Venereal Disease Information 27 (4)
(April 1946): 104-105.

Ducrey skin tests were conducted on 473 black hospital
patients. The researchers found that 29.5 percent of
the adult population tested showed positive skin
reactions. Positive skin reactions were found in none
of the 87 children tested. Also found that the
incidence of positive reactions began to occur between
the ages of fifteen and twenty-four. The positive skin
reactions occurred at an earlier age for females. As
expected, positive skin reactions occurred more
frequently in syphilitic individuals than in
nonsyphilitic individuals. The results of the study
cast serious doubt on the use of the Ducrey skin test as
a diagnostic tool. Positive results in over one-fourth
the black population tested may indicate a high
incidence of positive tests among patients with venereal
diseases other than syphilis.

260. Himes, Norman E. "Clinical Services for the Negro,"
Birth Control Review 16 (June 1932): 176-177.

The purpose of this study was to determine if clinical
services in the U.S. were reaching the black population.

It was proved that Negroes were being reached. In most
cases, the use of clinical services by blacks doubled
their population in communities that provided the
services.

261. Hindman, S. S. "Syphilis Among Insane Negroes," The
American Journal of Public Health 16 (August 1926):
218-224.

Uses data to draw attention to the prevalence of
syphilis in blacks in the South and emphasizes the
difficulty in getting a syphilitic black to take
treatment. Insufficient treatment results in acute
nervous conditions followed by general paralysis, tabes,
etc. Inherited syphilis and its possible effects for
several generations causes insanity in the black race as
well as the white race and is becoming an increasingly
important health issue in the South.

262. Hinton, Albert L. "Fighting Syphilis," Crisis 45 (5)
(May 1938):138-139, 146.

Describes the work of Dr. David Byrd in his public
clinic and his treatment of syphilis. Dr. Byrd served
as president of the National Medical Association in
1917-1918 and in 1938 was an advisor to its executive
board. Observes that syphilis "is responsible for more
than 10 percent of all insanity, 18 percent of all
diseases of the heart and blood vessels, for many of the
still births and the deaths of babies in the first weeks
of life." Dr. Byrd was appointed chairman of a national
commission whose purpose was to eradicate syphilis. Dr.
Byrd later became supervisor of the Public Clinic. Dr.
Byrd, with the assistance of an efficient staff of
workers including registered nurses, case workers, and
investigators, have taken a total of more than 18,000
blood tests at the facility in its five years of
existence. The procedure Dr. Byrd followed was: 1) find
the patient, 2) treat the patient until he is
non-infectious, and 3) prevent congenital syphilis.

263. Hoffman, Frederick L. "The Negro Health Problem,"
Opportunity 4 (April 1926): 119-121, 138.

Citing the great disparity between black morality and
birth rates and white morality and birth rates,
discusses issues "fundamental to the Negro health
problem." Among these are the reduction of immoral
sexual practices among blacks (responsiblity in part is
placed on the white man), housing (the elimination of
over-crowded and unsanitary conditions), the reduction
of infant mortality by educating mothers in pre-natal
and natal care, the systematic development of the body
(which suggests that the "Negro race" be taught to
breath properly and practice deep breathing daily and
considers Prohibition an event favorable to the health
of blacks), and better medical care (including more and
better facilities and more trained physicians and health
workers). Also discusses the increasing cases of mental

illness among blacks especially in the North which is
attributed to the increased strains of living in a more
industrial part of the country. Concludes by noting
that "one may safely conclude that the Negro is making
progress in health and disease resistance, but that
progress as yet falls far short of the corresponding
progress made by the white population."

264. Hoge, V. M. "What the Hospital Act Means to Negroes,"
National Negro Health News (April-June 1946):1.

The passage of the Hospital Survey and Construction Act
of 1946 showed the changing public attitude towards the
health of the nation with especially more attention to
blacks. Usually, the black community in the rural area
could not support a hospital. Blacks were served by the
community clinics which also provided emergency
services. The Hospital Act authorized $375 million to
help build hospitals nationwide. This grant-in-aid
program required that every dollar of Federal funds must
be met by $2 of State or local funds. It also required
that these hospitals must be maintained and operated
without federal help once they were built. A great
effort from State help was needed in achieving this
program. However, the Hospital Survey and Construction
Act had two purposes. First, it provided assistance to
the States in surveying overall State needs and in
making master plans for needed hospitals and health
centers. Second, it provided assistance for the
contruction necessary to carry out these plans.

265. Holland, Dorothy F. and Perrott, G. S. J. "Health of
the Negro," Milbank Memorial Fund Quarterly 16 (1938):5-38.

A summary of the studies of disabling illnesses based on
survey research. The first survey was conducted in New
York City in 1933. The second survey was conducted in
Atlanta, Cincinnati, Dallas, and Newark in 1935 and
1936. Includes a multitude of data based on the 170,000
responses to the two surveys. Most of the data pertain
to the incidences of disabling illnesses according to
race, sex, income group, occupational group, age, and
geographical location. The general findings are: (a)
blacks are 43 percent more likely than whites to be
struck by sickness that caused incapacitation for at
least one week; (b) on average, blacks are incapacitated
for eight days per year while whites are incapacitated
for five days per year; (c) black children are disabled
less than white children because of the lower incidences
of chronic disease in the former; (d) black adults are
more susceptible than whites to such chronic diseases as
pneumonia, cardiovascular-renal ailments, rheumatism,
and asthma; and (e) blacks who depended on public relief
experience twice as much disability as blacks who are
not on relief. Thus, it appears that low socioeconomic
status is more highly correlated with incidences of
chronic disease than are racial characteristics.

266.   Holmes, S. J.   "The Principle Causes of Death Among Negroes: A General Comparative Statement," Journal of Negro Education 6 (3) (July 1937): 289-302.

Examines the factors that affect the death rate of blacks and assumes that the birth rate of blacks will remain constant.   Argues that changes in the death rate will most likely affect the population of American blacks.   Views diseases which strike blacks before the close of the reproductive cycle as the most destructive. These diseases include: tuberculosis, the respiratory infections, venereal diseases, uterine cancer, the intestinal disorders of infancy, and puerperal fever. Rejects the argument that blacks are "constitutional inferior" and credits racism and poverty for the higher disease rate of blacks.

267.   Holoubek, J. E. and Holoubek, A. B.   "Heart Disease in the South: II. A Statistical Survey of One Hundred Seventeen Deaths Due to Rheumatic Heart Disease," American Heart Journal 34 (5) (November 1947): 709-714.

A study of 8,313 patients who were necropsied; 5,252 or 63.2 percent were blacks.   The series included 2,982 black men, 2,270 black women, 1,975 white men, and 1,086 white women.   Death was found to have been the result of heart disease in 1,045 patients.   In 117 cases, rheumatic heart disease was present.   This series of 117 subjects whose deaths were due to rheumatic heart disease has been analyzed according to sex, age and racial incidence, and the type of valvular involvement.

268.   Howles, James K.   "Sarcoidosis in the Negro," Southern Medical Journal 43 (7) (July 1950): 633-641.

Investigates the increase of death reports in blacks as a result of sarcoid infection.   Examines a number of cases in New Orleans where the infection is numerous. Discusses the terminology of the disease and develops two schools of thought.   Discusses the therapeutic measures and concludes that it can be treated to full recovery.   Presents several reasons why this disease has flourished among blacks and discusses the low resistance of the colored race to certain diseases.

269.   Hrdlicka, A.   "Full-Blooded American Negro," American Journal of Physical Anthropology 12 (July-September 1928):15-34.

The 1920s was a period during which scientific and pseudo-scientific studies of race and racial characteristics were popular.   This article, concentrating on the physical anthropological aspects of race, avoids some of the most blatant and offensive aspects of this sort of study, but is still an amazing document in social attitudes of the recent past.

270.   "Incidence of Syphilis Among Negroes in Washington," Journal of Social Hygiene 23 (June 1937): 330.

In 1933, Freedman's Hospital, Washington, admitted 4,982
patients to its wards; 11,743 patients were examined in
the clinics. Serologic examinations for syphilis were
made on 4,595 patients. The Neguchi modification of the
Wassermann test was used, including both
acetone-insoluble and cholesterinized antigens. Two,
three, and four plus readings were considered positive.
Of the 4,595 patients examined, an incidence of
serologic evidence of syphilis was found in 19.41
percent (or 892) - a much lower figure than other
figures reported in surveys of black hospital patients.
The highest percentage of syphilis was found in the
gynecologic clinic totalling 31.6 percent and the lowest
in the University health clinic - 7.9 percent of 38
students. The Wassermann reaction was positive in 27.7
percent of 610 pregnant women, and in 25.84 percent of
89 children in the age group 0-5 and in 13.3 percent of
68 children in the age group 6-10. The percentage for
the age groups 11-15, 16-20, 21-25 was 24 plus for each
group. The incidence seemed to be greater among the
lower socio-economic levels. Twenty-six percent of 183
unmarried girls under the age of 20 gave a positive
reaction for syphilis. Excluding the pregnant women,
the incidence among females was not extremely higher
than males.

271.   "Infant Mortality Among Negroes in New York City,"
American Journal of Public Health 22 (December 1932):1295.

A study of the black infant mortality rate in New York
City. The rate averaged 209 per 1,000 live births in
the years 1910-14, and 104 during the period 1927-32.
Infant death rate among blacks is almost double that
among the population of New York City as a whole.
Control measures, therefore, need to be concentrated on
areas of the city with large black populations.
Tuberculosis causes an undue proportion of deaths of
black children. Their death rate from this disease is
four times the city rate. In infant deaths due to
malformations, the rate is actually lower among blacks
than it is in the entire population. The death rate
from puerperal causes among black infants was 8 per
1,000 live births in 1923.

272.   Jackson, Algernon B.   "The Need of Health Education
Among Negroes," Opportunity 2 (20) (August 1924): 235-236.

Stresses the need for health education among blacks.
Observes that there is a very vital and definite need to
educate whites to understand that the question of health
is a national rather than a racial one, which demands
national consideration and treatment, or our whole
scheme for human betterment breaks down. In a report
from the Surgeon General of the United States Army, it
was found that physically, blacks are better than the
white man, but they still have a higher morbidity and
mortality rate. Attributes this to no other reason than
blacks' general ignorance and indifference regarding the
rules of health and self-preservation. Suggests that

the focus of civic, state and nation organizations
should be the education of all classes of persons of all
races, especially to those groups hampered by social,
economic, and general living restrictions. Concludes
with a phrase of Booker T. Washington, "Without health,
and until we reduce the high death rate, it will be
impossible for us to have permanent success in business,
in property getting, in acquiring education, or to show
other evidences of progress. Without health and long
life, all else fails."

273. Jackson, N. C. "Community Organization Activities
Among Negroes for Venereal Disease Control," Social Forces 23
(October 1944): 65-70.

Discusses Social Protection Committees at work in
several communities in the Southeast that seek to
interest blacks in the problems of venereal disease and
efforts toward eradication. These committees are
working closely with other groups and organizations and
appear to be making considerable progress. Several
factors contribute to this progress: (1) planning and
undertaking activities as part of overall community
development; (2) stimulating and enlisting the
involvement of black groups and organizations; and (3)
providing assistance to the groups own activity rather
than for it.

274. Jackson, N. C. "Social Protection Among Negroes,"
Journal of Social Hygiene 31 (5) (May 1945): 276-283.

A report of a meeting designed to interest rural groups
in a social protection program, particularly black
participation in attacking venereal disease in Region
VII on four points: Law Enforcement, Health, Welfare and
Prevention, and Education. Region VII consisted of the
states of Tennessee, South Carolina, Mississippi,
Georgia, Florida and Alabama which accounts for one
third of the venereal disease infections of the nation.
Figures show that prevalence was 309.4 per one thousand
blacks and 40.7 per one thousand whites (the highest
rate in the nation for any area). Suggests that these
findings show that within the same geographic region,
wherever a rate is high for one racial group, it is also
high in another racial group. Two factors which makes
the job of reducing venereal disease difficult lies in
the economic conditions in the area and the racial
composition of the citizens in the area. This is
significant because wherever unfavorable economic
conditions exists, there are high sickness rates, low
educational standards and reduced government services
for the citizens' welfare. Mississippi, South Carolina,
Alabama, Georgia, and Tennessee ranked lowest in per
capita income payments in the United States,
respectively. In reference to racial composition,
blacks make up large proportions of the state's
population; ranging from 17.4 percent in Tennessee to
49.2 percent in Mississippi. Because more than 50
percent of the South's black population lives in this

area, it is paramount that the citizens support efforts
to eliminate venereal disease.

275. Johnson, Bascom. "Venereal Disease Health Education
Project for Negroes in Texas," Journal of Social Hygiene 30
(2) (February 1944): 72-76.

The American Social Health Association authorized Bascom
Johnson, Director of the Association in Texas, to invite
seven black selectees to serve as an Advisory and
Sponsoring Committee for the Venereal Disease Health
Education Project for blacks in Texas. The founding of
this project resulted from concern with venereal disease
because of the large number of black selectees whom were
rejected by the Navy, Army, and auxilliary services
because they had syphilis and gonorrhea. Each selectee
was employed for a three month trial period (Summer) to
conduct an intensive health education project among
blacks on the nature, causes, kinds, spread, and cure of
the venereal disease. Projects included four motion
picture films of the Association entitled: "With These
Weapons," "Health is a Victory," "Plain Facts," and "In
Defense of the Nation." The group included ministers,
beauty culturists, insurance agents, labor groups,
women's organizations, young people's groups, and summer
schools and college campuses. The Negro Sponsoring
Committee under the direction of Mr. Toles carried out
planned projects and reported their findings to a group
of Army, Navy, Public Health Officials, Federal and
State officials. The unanimous decision was to
continue.

276. Johnson, Cernoria D. "Fort Worth, Texas, Negro Health
Center." National Negro Health News 14 (1) (1946): 7-11.

The establishment of the Carver Health Center for blacks
in Fort Worth, Texas had its beginning in the health
work started in the community shortly after World War I.
Reverend F. Rivers Barnwell was the first black lay
health worker employed by the state health agency to
organize and direct a black health program. He started
the Volunteer Health League movement which became a
state-wide influence in the promotion of a sound health
education program. The League cooperated with the City
Health Department, as the blacks in the area decided to
solve their own health problems through their own
efforts. The Carver Health Center was furnished and
equipped through the generous donations from citizens
and their organizations. The City Health Department
financed the cost of utilities, medicines, and supplies,
and a full-time registered nurse who supervised the
center. Through this kind of community organization,
civic pride and social consciousness are aroused, and
many gains are made for the general community welfare.

277. Johnson, Charles S. "Dentistry and Negro Health,"
Opportunity 5 (10) (October 1927): 287-288.

The new importance of dentistry as a vital health
service, over its earlier status as a mere mechanical
art, is revealing more of the glaring inadequacies in
the care of black health. A reference is made to
Bulletin 19 of the Carnegie Foundation for the
Advancement of Teaching on Dental Education in the
United States and Canada, which gives the results of a
five year study by William J. Gies, who devoted a
chapter to dental training for blacks. The emphasis is
on the deficiency of dental service for blacks. Notes
that of the 70,000 dental practitioners in the United
States, only about 1,300 are black. The inadequate
number of black dentists indicates a tendency to
restrict the number of black students in the mixed
schools which adds to the gravity of the situation.
Recommends the establishment of fellowship and loan
funds at the best institutions to support the education
of selected blacks as practitioners, teachers or
investigators to solve the problem of adequate
production and uniform distribution of black physicians,
surgeons, dentists and nurses. This would also provide
leadership in all divisions of health service for
blacks.

278. Johnson, Charles S. "New Trends in Negro Mortality,"
Opportunity 2 (22) (October 1924): 290-291.

Disturbed by what seemed to be complacency on the part
of blacks since an announcement in 1923 that the life
span of blacks had increased and the death rate
materially decreased. Argues that health improvement
follows a stern law which tolerates no relaxation from
vigilance and points out that although deaths from
tuberculosis, against which the greatest health efforts
had been directed, showed a slight decrease, there had
been sharp increases in deaths from diseases incidental
to pregnancy and childbirth, from cancer, and from
pneumonia. In all of these, there had been a steady
decline among whites. The diseases which showed
pronounced increases were those which had been
unwatched.

279. Johnson, Charles S. "Mortality of Negro Mothers,"
Opportunity 3 (28) (April 1925): 99.

The problem of the increasing mortality among black
women at childbirth is discussed. The Federal Census
mortality figures released in 1923 showed that the rate
of deaths for black mothers in Kentucky was 15.4 per
1,000 as compared to 5.4 for white mothers, 12.2 in
South Carolina against 7.4 for white mothers, in
Mississippi 10.9 as compared with 6.6, in North Carolina
10.7 against 6.7. These deaths were found to be most
common among mothers who are forced to work and where
proper medical care cannot be secured. Also presents
data that show the large number of black women forced to
labor.

280.   Johnson, Charles S.   "The Socio-Economic Background of
Negro Health Status," The Journal of Negro Education 18
(Summer 1949):   429-435.

Begins by emphasizing the unbreakable link between
socio-economic factors and health status, the latter
being hindered by the former. Discusses the current
effects of the economic status of blacks on health under
incomes and occupations, housing and illiteracy and
superstition. The low economic status of most blacks is
"a causative factor in ill-health" both because of the
inability of the poor black to afford good medical
attention and the inability to afford a standard of
living conductive to good health. Observes that the
occupations in which blacks find themselves are
generally more hazardous and strenuous which affects
life-expectancy. Although the recent war postively
affected black occupations, their relative position in
the labor force changed little. Low income necessitates
poor housing, another major contributing factor to poor
health. Obsolete dwellings which require a great deal
of repair are conducive to unsanitary conditions which
are in turn linked to the spread of disease. Segregated
residential areas prevent those blacks who are able from
enhancing their dwelling status. Finally, illiteracy
and superstition (both due to lack of proper education)
prevent blacks from seeking the kinds of medical
attention necessary for health status improvement.
Ignorant blacks fall back on hear-say remedies for
illnesses readily curable by medical means. In
conclusion, stresses that it is in the best interest of
all the nation to work toward socio-economic equality
since in the premature loss of a black citizen, the
community loses both a consumer and a producer.

281.   Jones, Eugene Kinckle.   "The Negro's Struggle for
Health," Opportunity 1 (6) (June 1923): 4-5.

Research into the conditions of black health in Africa
and in slavery in America indicates that it was to the
advantage of the masters to keep their slaves in good
health. Data showing the death rates of the white and
black populations of southern cities during the
mid-1800's indicate that the white death rate was far in
excess of that of blacks. Notes that at the close of
the Civil War, a group of blacks living principally in
the rural South, possessed relatively good health and
were prepared with a good physical background to begin a
life of freedom and to take up the difficult problems of
a new civilization. Explores the struggle of blacks in
seeking social equality in acquiring more adequate and
healthful surroundings in the city to combat diseases
which result from a poor environment.

282.   Jones, H. Leonard, Jr., Wetzel, Frederick E. and Black,
Boyd K. "Sickle Cell Anemia with Striking
Electrocardiographic Abnormalities and Other Unusual Features
with Autopsy," Annals of Internal Medicine 29 (July-December
1948): 928-935.

A report of a 22 year old black who was admitted to a Naval Hospital in 1946, 11 hours after the onset of a severe substernal chest pain. This case of sickle cell anemia with autopsy is considered worthy of reporting because of gross electrocardiographic changes, even though quickly but partially reversible after the hemolytic crises, led researchers to expect marked myocardial damage. The autopsy revealed only simple hypertrophy and moderate interstitual edema. The patient also had a coexisting dueodenal ulcer which was a confusing element in the clinical picture. The weight of his spleen was 5 grams, the second smallest reported in the literature.

283.   Jones, R. Frank and Price, Kline A.   "The Incidence of Gonorrhea Among Negroes," The Journal of Negro Education 6 (1937): 364-392.

The authors note that gonorrhea is a disease that afflicts both blacks and whites. The main difference regarding gonorrhea among the races is the fact that whites seek treatment more often than blacks. The authors cite an appalling lack of education regarding this disease among blacks. Blacks are not taught that chemical solutions and condoms can treat and prevent gonorrhea. Blacks are not afforded an education which would show that the disease is easily spread, particularly through prostitution. The authors note that in each 1,000 person segment of society, blacks suffer five more cases of gonorrhea than whites. Education regarding gonorrhea is essential if the black affliction rate is to be reduced--the same education afforded to whites.

284.   Jordan, Weymouth T.   "Plantation Medicine in the Old South," Alabama Review 3 (1950):83-107.

A historical literature review of plantation health. Notes that blacks were given inadequate health care in the ante-bellum period. However, it was also the case that slaveowners realized the personal economic disaster that could result if slaves were too ill to work. Therefore, whites had an incentive to at least administer "home remedies" to black slaves. Slaveowners often had "medical chests" full of paraphernalia. In addition, black females were often given training in the use of medicine, "home remedies," and procedures that would prevent diseases. These black females would often serve as "nurses" for slave and master alike. Textbooks documenting black illnesses were nonexistent, but agricultural journals and general publications did contain medical information to help in the treatment of slaves. Describes the writings of John Wilson, a doctor concerned with black health care. Wilson wrote several pamphlets which were never published in book form. Some of Wilson's titles include "The Peculiarities and Diseases of Negroes," and "The Negro-His Diet, Clothing, etc.", "The Negro-His Mental and Moral Peculiarities" and "Matrimonial Alliances of Negroes." In short, what

little medical information concerning blacks did exist
in ante-bellum times was a conglomeration of good advice
and racist propaganda.

285. Karlan, K. C. "A Comparative Study of Psychoses Among
Negroes and Whites in the New York State Prisons."
Psychiatric Quarterly 13 (1939):160-164.

Reports that the incidence of psychoses in the general
population is higher in blacks than in whites. Studies
blacks and whites at New York State prisons and
concludes that the incidence of functional psychoses
among black inmates is about the same as that among
white prisoners. Blacks have, therefore, no racial
predisposition to mental disease. High incidence of
mental disease among blacks is probably due to cultural,
social and economic causes. Observes that the
incidences of psychoses among prison inmates is five to
ten times as high as that of the general population.

286. Katz, Sol, Hussey, Hugh H. and Walsh, Bernard J.
"Syphilitic Heart Disease Probably Due to Congenital
Syphilis: Report of Two Cases," Annals of Internal Medicine
22 (January-June 1945): 606-614.

Reports of case studies of syphilitic heart disease. In
one case Wassermann or Kahn tests of the mother's blood
or of the umbilical cord blood were not made. One five
and a half year old South Carolina, black girl, was
admitted to Children's Hospital, Washington, D.C.,
because of acute pyelitis. Upon exam the heart was
recorded as normal. Wassermann test were also negative.
Later upon admission in 1939 to Gallinger Municipal
Hospital, she was diagnosed as having syphilitic heart
disease and blindness by age eleven. A loud systolic
murmur was heard at the cardiac apex and in the aortic
area to the right of the sternum. Upon her last
admission August 10, 1941 on her eighth day she became
very dyspneic and cyanotic. There were frequent
premature beats and numerous rates at the bases of both
lungs. She died after the onset of acute distress at
age 22. Another 12 year old black female was admitted
on March 28, 1929 with the complaint of syspnea. Later
died April 9, 1929. A review of her record at
Children's Hospital revealed that she was a full term
baby. She was said to have been "purple" at birth, and
bled from the nose for four days. She had been admitted
for chaffing of the buttocks. Seven years later,
examination in the outpatient department showed
Wassermann strongly positive. Antiosyphilitic therapy
was begun June 14, 1924. On August 23, 1924 she was
readmitted because she was not doing well. She died on
the twenty-first hospital day. Postmortem examination
showed marked enlargement of the heart, particularly to
the left. When the heart was opened, all chambers were
found to be dilated. Both lungs were moderately
congested and edematous. The pathological diagnosis was
syphilitic heart disease.

287. Kittrell, Flemmie P. "The Negro Family as a Health
Agency," Journal of Negro Education 18 (1949): 422-428.

The author contends that the family is the most
important agency in health care. Constructive early
years are said to be essential to the development of
living patterns which will contribute to good health
throughout life. However, blacks often lack
constructive formative years because both parents must
work to provide income. Thus, it is more difficult for
black children to receive good guidance early in life.
The author discusses the subtle negative effects that
segregation and discrimination can have on the
development and health of blacks. Argues that the
structure and composition of the house, its furnishings,
interpersonal relationships, and food are the major
points around which health revolves. Emphasizes that
children must receive the proper education regarding
these components if they are to enjoy good health. They
must learn how to properly feed, clothe, and house
themselves if they are to be healthy, and the family has
the responsibility to impart the proper education in
these matters to children. Contends that blacks need
greater economic security, a greater appreciation of
home living, and a more focused effort on helping black
children to secure general education if blacks are to
improve their health status.

288. Knox, J. H. Mason et al. "The Health Problem of the
Negro Child," American Journal of Public Health 16 (August
1926):805-9.

Explores reasons why some black children are in
generally poorer health than most white children. The
major question that the author seeks to answer is "Are
the deplorable health conditions among the Negroes
inherent, and due to racial inferiority or to
difficulties of adaptation and acclimatization? Or are
they the result of environmental and, therefore,
preventable factors?" There was a reduction in the
white infant mortality rate from 1915 to 1922 of
twenty-six percent and in the colored infant mortality
rate for the same period of thirty-nine percent. It is
recognized, however, that it is easier to reduce an
infant mortality rate which starts high (black) than to
further reduce a comparatively low rate (white). Among
the causes of mortality among black infants,
tuberculosis, syphilis, and pneumonia are conspicuous.
Twenty percent of all deaths under one year among blacks
are the result of either tuberculosis, syphilis, or
diseases of the respiratory tract, but only ten percent
of deaths of white infants are due to the same causes.
The incidence of venereal diseases among black children
is significant. Some 9.5 percent of black children gave
a positive Wassermann reaction. Concludes with the
opinion that excessive black infant mortality is due to
the lower economic status of blacks and to lower
standards of morals and education.

289. "Late Neurosyphilis in North American Negroes and
Whites," The Journal of Venereal Disease Information 26 (12)
(December 1945): 267.

Clinical and postmortem results of representative groups
of black and white hospital patients with late
neurosyphilis are examined. Attempts to determine the
incidence and trend of general paresis in the black and
white population. The results indicate that general
paresis is directly related to the syphilis ratio, with
no difference in relative general paresis incidence
between blacks and whites. The onset of general paresis
occurred earlier in blacks due to earlier infection by
the syphilitic infection. The incidence of general
paresis was highest among black women. Stationary
paresis in whites tends to be more chronic and
prolonged. The results also indicate that tabes
dorsalis in all its varieties occur with the same
frequency among blacks as among whites. Concludes that
organic psychosis due to meningovascular syphilis
combined with other diseases occur more frequently among
blacks.

290. Lee, Isabel A. "Health Education Among Negroes, Coahoma
County, Misssissippi," National Negro Health News 16 (2)
(April-June 1948): 9-11.

Describes the success in four areas of health education
in Coahoma County, Mississippi where 77 percent of the
62,000 residents are black. First, teachers were
provided with an in-service training program heightening
their awareness of health problems and solutions.
Second, a health inventory list was distributed to
schools and teachers which was later evaluated showing
improvements in school environments, sanitary use of
toilets, lunches and the number of student health
referrals. Third, the activities of community health
clubs have provided leadership in health education and
performed health related services to the community and
have solicited the support of ministers and other
influential leaders or groups in the service of health
education. Finally, maternal and child health clinics
are held to reach pre-school children, their mothers and
midwives. Other clinics cover other health topics such
as venereal and communicable diseases, immunization and
even guidance clinics for handicapped children were
held. Concludes by noting that joint planning and
cooperation by all persons and groups involved is the
"keynote" to the effectiveness of health education in
Coahoma County.

291. Leider, M., Brookins, S., and McDaniel, V. "Biography
of a Civilian Committee on Venereal Disease Control," Journal
of Social Hygiene 30 (2) (February 1944): 67-72.

A report of the conception, birth and early development
of the War-Time Negro Committee on Venereal Disease
Control, organized by the authors in November 1943. The
town of Pensacola, Florida abuts a large Naval Air

Station. About 25 percent of the civilian army
population is black, with only 4 percent of the military
black. An increase of 15 percent black strength is
expected. With an anticipated increase in black
soldiers, a runaway situation of venereal disease was
feared. In November 1943, preliminary meetings were
held with a small group of black residents, military
personnel, and civic-minded lay persons to discuss the
nature of the venereal disease control problems. Among
those who responded was a representative of the National
Association for the Advancement of Colored People
(NAACP), the principal of Booker T. Washington High
School, two black physicians, two ministers, the black
investigator of the county health department, several
black merchants and businessmen and others. After
parliamentary procedures had been affected, the
formulation and implementation of a program of action
was adopted as feasible for the immediate and remote
future and adapted to local conditions. In a period of
three months, a significant record of accomplishment was
made. Shortly, thereafter, the organization expanded to
include most of the black professionals, a large
percentage of ministers, several teachers, and a large
number of lay people of both sexes.

292. Leider, M. "Civilian Committees on Venereal Disease
Control - A Progress Note," Journal of Social Hygiene 31
(1945): 441-448.

A report on a civilian committee on V.D. control (The
Negro Wartime Health Committee of Pensacola, Florida).
Written by a Lieutenant Commander of the U.S. Navy.
Provides a brief history of the Committee as well as a
synopsis of the activities and accomplishments since the
groups inception (November, 1943). The synopsis
includes a discussion of the Health Committee's
membership growth, fund raising, headquarter locating
and projects. The second half of the article focuses on
the establishment of a similar organization by white
citizens of Pensacola, the Gulf Health and Welfare
Council. Included is the group's charter, general
objectives, and immediate objectives. Also discusses
the Council's significant accomplishments during the six
months since its inception.

293. Lenroot, Katherine F. "The Health-Education Program of
the Children's Bureau, With Particular Reference to Negroes,"
Journal of Negro Education 6 (1937):506-12.

Legislation was passed in 1912 for the formation of a
Children's Bureau in the Department of Commerce and
Labor. The Bureau was utilized to study problems
relating to mothers and children. In 1936, however, the
Children's Bureau became an arm of far-reaching change
under the Social Security Act. Research is conducted in
Child Development, Industrial, Social Service,
Delinquency, and Statistical Research. Not only is the
Children's Bureau in charge of research, but educational
material is handed out and health care is available

through the Children's Bureau. Drawing from other works
which highlight the special problems of health care for
black children, the author emphasizes the necessity of
providing health care to blacks through the Children's
Bureau. According to federal consultants, the
Children's Bureau has succeeded in bringing such care to
black children. In addition, the Children's Bureau has
committed itself to developing postgraduate courses for
Southern blacks so that black physicians can bring more
and better services to the black community. The author,
the Chief of the Children's Bureau, believes that a
higher level of funding and the continued support of the
federal and state governments will allow the Children's
Bureau to do even more for whites and blacks alike.

294. Leopold, Eugene J. "Diabetes in the Negro Race,"
Annals of Internal Medicine 5 (1931-32): 285-293.

Verifies that diabetes mellitus is not an uncommon
disease among blacks. For example, the death rate of
diabetes mellitus in Baltimore in 1930 was 28.02 for
white persons and 30.01 for blacks per hundred thousand
inhabitants. White deaths from diabetes were 2.36
percent of all deaths and black deaths were 0.96
percent. Among new admissions to the Outpatient
Department of Johns Hopkins Hospital blacks formed 31.9
percent and 28.8 percent of the new admissions to the
Diabetic Clinic. Diabetes is even more common among
black females than in the white race. Overall diabetes
in blacks is not different in any way from the disease
as found among whites.

295. Lewis, J. H. The Biology of the Negro (Chicago: The
University of Chicago Press, 1942).

The introduction of this book is brief, but with clear
content and purpose. The subject matter is arranged
under following chapter headings: Population and Vital
Statistics; Anatomy of the Negro; Biochemical and
Physiological Characteristics; Medical Diseases:
Surgical Diseases; Obstetrics and Gynecology; Diseases
of the Skin; Diseases of the Eye, Ear, Nose, and Throat;
and Dental Diseases. There is a complete index of
authors and subject index. This comment upon the
interest and merit of the book is quoted: "when a
balance is struck between the assets and liabilities of
the Negro is his struggle with the environment, which
includes diseases, it is found to be in his favor. This
is expressed in his ability not only to survive, but to
flourish on two continents." Differentiating between
biological and environment factors in diseases, the
author examines the greatest liabilities of the Negro--
his excessive morbidity and mortality rates from heart
disease, tuberculosis, and syphilis. He suggests that
the two last-mentioned diseases are more virulent in
Negroes because they are four hundred or more years
younger in them than in white people. "The Negro's
assets are his birth rate, his physical stamina, and his

resistance to malaria, exanthemata, and certain surgical conditions."

296. Lewis, Julian. "Number and Geographic Location of Negro Physicians in the United States," Journal of the American Medical Association 104 (14) (April 11, 1935):1272-1273.

A compilation of data regarding the location of black physicians in the United States in 1932. About 10 percent of the population of the country is black, but only 2.5 percent of the physicians are black - one physician for every three thousand blacks. Although most of the black population lives in the South, the majority of the black physicians lives in the North. Yet most black physicians graduated from southern medical schools. Black physicians tend to concentrate in large cities regardless of the size of the black population in that city.

297. Lewis, Stephen J. "The Negro in the Field of Dentistry," Opportunity 2 (19) (July 1924): 207.

A brief historic background of blacks' advances in the dental field along with a description of the difficulties and limitations that gave little hope of hurried accomplishment. Explains that as late as 1880 there were fewer than a dozen legal black dental practitioners. Most of those who had entered the profession had done so largely through suggestions or urged by white practitioners for whom they had been employed as laboratory assistants coupled with the desire of white dentists to dispose of black patients. Consequently, the element of selective choice of a professional career as such played only a minor in blacks entering the field of dentistry. Describes the economic and psychological problems faced by the pioneers and their perserverance in contributing to the establishment, growth, and expansion of two black dental colleges.

298. Lingberg, D. O. N. "Chest Roetgen-Ray Study of the Adult Negro Population of an Entire Community," Annals of Internal Medicine 8 (1934-35): 1421-1426.

Attempts to determine whether tuberculosis in blacks could be controlled using the same methods employed for the white population. The adult black population of Macon County, Illinois (1933-34) was studied. The Roetgen-Ray survey was conducted on a large scale. Single chest films were made on 1,005 out of 1,232 adults, or a percentage of 81.6. All ages between 20 and 94 years were examined in the survey. The examinations were made in nearly equal proportions between the sexes. The results lead to the suggestion that tuberculosis in blacks may be controlled by the same methods that are being successfully employed for the white population in as much as the disease in blacks appears to be dependent upon the same factors of economic standards, undue exposure to infection and environment. As a result, education and adequate provision of sanitorium beds in diagnostic facilities have served importantly to reduce the morbidity and mortality among the racial group.

299. Martin, Collier. "Stricture of the Rectum," Journal of the American Medical Association 101 (27) (November 11, 1933):1550-1552.

Discusses the disease of stricture of the anus and it's peculiarity to blacks, especially black females. After extensive study of 169 cases, notes that the disease is common to blacks simply because of racial susceptibility. The disease presents itself in the female as a stricture whereas in the male, it is more of a sore on the genitals. Points out that there is no known cure and the best course of treatment is either a proctotomy and eventually a permanent colostomy. Concludes with abstracts of discussions by different physicians of various stricture cases.

300. Martin, Ralph G. "Doctor's Dream in Harlem," New Republic 114 (June 3, 1946):798-800.

Discusses the need for Lafargue Clinic, a psychiatric clinic in Harlem run by Dr. Frederic Wertham. The white psychiatrist started the clinic because he felt that psychoanalysis and psychotherapy were not the private property of the rich, but the common property of the people. He dubbed his treatment program "social psychiatry," which meant understanding a patient's economic and community life as well as his sex life before he could treat him properly. A compelling reason to start up this clinic was the fact that juvenile delinquency in Harlem reached a high of fifty-three percent of the city total. Notes that many people balked at the idea of a single clinic to serve the 400,000 blacks in Harlem. Dr. Wertham stated it was a success, however, because all types of individuals were being served.

301. Mason, Ulysses G. "Problems Incidental to Negro Staff Training in Hospitals," Hospitals 3 (March 1944):71-72.

Lack of hospital facilities is the chief problem facing the practicing black physicians. Those hospitals affording hospital facilities to black doctors produce the best qualified and trained black physicians and surgeons. Since there are countless numbers of facilities which do not provide such access, many black physicians fail to ever reach their full intellectual potential. Admission of black physicians to these hospitals would be the ideal and democratic way of meeting this problem. But the major obstacles include lack of hospitals willing to participate and the fact of racial intolerance. If black physicians are kept from the main flow of new medical advances, both the white and black sick population will suffer.

302. Massey, Estelle G.   "What is a Nurse?" Opportunity 12
(2) (February 1934): 52-53.

Discusses the public's misconceptions and unfamiliarity
with the black nurse and her place in the social order.
Notes three areas which may be responsible for negative
attitudes and status of the black nurse. First, the
type of schools which have been created for training,
rather than educating nurses. Second, the type of
student to whom this training has been given. Third,
the people who have been responsible for this training.
Concludes that the nurse needs to be interpreted anew in
most communities. No matter how much it may try, the
community cannot overlook the service rendered by the
nurse. If the public insists upon and helps to provide
for the proper education of the nurse, it may expect a
highly specialized worker whose contribution to the
general welfare of the community will more than
compensate for the effort and cost of educating her.

303. Massey-Riddle, Estelle G.   "The Training and Placement
of Negro Nurses," Journal of Negro Education (1936):42-43.

Discusses the problems of black nurses. After
completion of training, black nurses are ostracized by
others in the profession as not being capable of
performing their tasks. However, since hospital
administrators have discovered that it is more
economical for a young nurse to care for the sick than
older, more experienced nurses, many black, beginning
nurses are being hired at lower wages to help fill the
need.

304. Mathis, Annie Maie.   "Negro Public Health Nursing in
Texas," Southern Workman 55 (July 1927): 302-303.

This article examines the activities of the State Public
Negro Nurse in Texas. There is a need for such a person
and it continues to grow. She goes into the black
community and organizes people in order to train them so
that they will be able to learn vital health skills.
She also reports on the deplorable conditions that cause
diseases and deaths, and how "clean-up weeks" attempt to
resolve this kind of situation. She not only gives
adult and pre-natal classes, but also, along with a
delegation of fellow Negro nurses, attends conferences.
There they learn new techniques and suggestions which
they take back to their communities and put them in
effect.

305. Maund, Alfred. "New Day Dawning." Opportunity 24
(January, 1946): 206-207.

Summary findings of a survey mailed to 42,500 white
doctors listed in the A.M.A. Directory concerning
segregation/discrimination in medical and hospital care.

306. Maxwell, C. H. and Pennell, Maryland Y. "Health
Services in Negro Schools of Less than College Grade,"
Journal of Negro Education 18 (1949): 418-421.

Presents the results of a nationwide study of child
health services conducted by the American Academy of
Pediatrics. The study indicates that where there is
segregation of white and non-white students (17 states
and the District of Columbia), there is less extensive
school medical service that there is in other parts of
the country. However, the data reveal that black and
white students apparently receive equal school health
care. The findings also show that the medical personnel
who work in the schools in the Southeastern United
States (where black population is greatest) are
predominantly employed by the official health agency of
the area rather than by the official education agency.
This pattern is reversed in the remainder of the nation.

307. Maxwell, U. S. and Wakeham, Glen. "The Basal Metabolic
Rate of the American Negro, With Particular Reference to the
Effect of Menstruation on the Female," Journal of American
Medical Association 29 (January-June 1945): 223-226.

A study of the basal metabolic rate of black women
during the menstrual cycle to determine if the values of
the black woman differs from the standard value for
white North Americans to suggest a racial factor in
basal metabolism. Twenty-seven women between the ages
of 17 and 35 were studied. The tests were carried out
in a metabolism laboratory and were made before, during
and after menstruation with an average interval of seven
days. Tests were also conducted on 14 men between the
ages of 18 and 24 years old. Concludes that black women
have a lower basal metabolic rate than the value
reported for white women. There appears to be a
pre-menstrual rise in basal metabolism with a lowering
during actual menstruation and in the immediate
post-menstrual period. Yet, the basal metabolic rate of
black women is not significantly lower than those of
white subjects.

308. McCreary, A. B. "Control of Typhoid in Richmond
County, North Carolina," Journal of the American Medical
Association 97 (14) (October 3, 1931):998-999.

A description of the methods used to eradicate typhoid
fever in Richmond County, N.C., where 40 percent of the
county was black and 99 percent of them were not
immunized. The health officer elicited the aid of the
black clergy and made a presentation that if they were
to be consistently religious, they must take pains to
protect their body from disease. This was successful
and led to black children being vaccinated against
smallpox. In these talks, good screens, safe sewage
disposal, pure water and milk supplies were stressed.
The approach was viewed as successful because the
typhoid rate decreased strikingly.

309.   "Medical Education for Negro Students," Journal of the American Medical Association 80 (25) (June 23, 1923):1856.

An editorial noting the inadequacy of facilities for education of black physicians, dentists, pharmacists, nurses and the lack of these professionals in practice. Problem is partly attributed to lack of funds to provide adequate training to all qualified students who apply. Notes that the two schools who are moderately well equipped to furnish education in medicine, pharmacy and dentistry, Howard University and Meharry Medical College, can accept one third or one fourth of the qualified applicants. These two training facilities have Foundations offering large funds upon the condition they secure corresponding funds from alumni and friends. Observes that these institutions are worthy of consideration by those who have money to give.

310.   "Medical Education in the United States," Journal of the American Medical Association 87 (8) (August 21, 1926):565-583.

Page 573 presents a brief discussion of "Negro Medical Students and Graduates". It was included in the paper "owing to the special interest that has been shown recently in regard to the numbers of black medical students." A table lists the medical schools, the number of black medical students enrolled and the number of black graduates for the 1923-1924, 1924-1925 and 1925-1926 sessions.

311.   "Medical Education in the United States," Journal of the American Medical Association 89 (8) (August 20, 1927):601-610.

Page 608 presents a discussion and table of the number of black medical students enrolled in the various medical schools. For the 1926-1927 session there was a total of 526 black medical students and 126 graduates.

312.   "Medical Education in the United States," Journal of the American Medical Association 91 (7) (August 18, 1928):473-481.

Page 479 includes a discussion and table presentation of the number of black medical students and number of graduates for the 1927-28 session, by medical school. For 1927-28 there were 530 black students and 123 graduates.

313.   "Medical Education in the United States," Journal of the American Medical Association 97 (9) (August 29, 1931):611-628.

Page 624 includes a discussion entitled "Negroes in Medical Schools" and presents a summary and table of the number of black medical students and graduates by medical school. For the session 1927-1928 there were 510 black medical students and 120 graduates. For the

1930-31 session, there were 504 black medical students
and 114 graduates.

314. "Medical Education in the United States," Journal of
the American Medical Association 99 (9) (August 27,
1932):731-746.

Page 741 includes a discussion entitled "Negroes in
Medical Schools" with a summary and table of the number
of black medical students and graduates in the medical
schools. In the 1931-32 session there were 479 black
medical students and 122 graduates.

315. "Ministers Plan Health Institute." Atlantic Daily
World. Cited in National Negro Health News 14 (3) (1946):
24.

Atlanta's black ministers, aroused by the high
tuberculosis rate among the people of their race, held a
2 day health institute in Atlanta on September 25 and
26. The institute was arranged in cooperation with the
Negro branch of the Atlanta Tuberculosis Association.
Reverend Harry V. Richardson, chaplain at Tuskegee
Institute, Alabama, and Dr. W. Montague Cobb, professor
at Howard University, Washington, D.C., were among those
who attended.

316. Mitchell, A. Graeme and Cook, William C. "Mongolism in
the Negro," Journal of the American Medical Association 99
(25) (December 17, 1932):2105-2106.

Discusses four cases of mongolism in blacks to document
its occurrence. Each case includes a history,
diagnostic information and photographs.

317. Mitchell, Isadore C. "Will Socialized Dentistry Solve
the Problem?" Opportunity 12 (2) (February 1934): 51, 64.

This essay is a reply to Lester B. Granger's article,
"The Negro Physician and Socialized Medicine," which
appeared in the December 1933 issue of Opportunity. Dr.
Mitchell asks, "What class of Negroes is in need of
socialized dentistry?" He suggests that it is not the
wealthy blacks for they will not consent to receive
wholesale dental service by dentists whom they do not
personally select; it is not the indigent for they have
no choice and they usually receive free service from the
County; it is the middle class black with not quite
enough money to pay for efficient dental service.
Argues that if the object of socialized dentistry is to
relieve pain, cure diseases, and restore lost organs in
whole or in part by dentists assigned to specific
communities, it will partly solve the problem. The
science of dentistry has for its principal objects the
educating of the public so that it will not be necessary
to restore the dental organs, but if it is necessary,
will do so efficiently. Proposes that organized
dentistry must solve the problem because it seeks to
educate; to prevent diseases; and to correct and

maintain dental health through physical and mental means.

318. Mitchell, Martha Carolyn. "Health and the Medical Profession in the Lower South, 1845-1860," Journal of Southern History 10 (1944):424-46.

Equates the ante-bellum South with a newly settled frontier. The lower South (Alabama, Mississippi, Georgia, and Louisiana) contained few physicians, little medicine, poor food, and, in many cases, inadequate housing. Blacks, as members of an entrenched underclass, were especially susceptible to disease. Yellow fever and cholera outbreaks became epidemics on a number of occasions in coastal regions from 1845 to 1860. Morbidity and mortality rates were very high for blacks. Part of the problem for blacks stemmed from the fact that southern doctors believed that blacks were especially susceptible to some diseases and immune from others. For both blacks and whites, doctors could only treat diseases on a hit-or-miss basis because there was not a consensus on the causes of most diseases. Nevertheless, this time period saw new ideas being raised concerning contagion, germ theory, and insect theory. The groundwork was laid for future improvements.

319. Montagu, M. F. A. "The Physical Anthropology of the American Negro," Psychiatry 7 (1) (February 1944): 31-44.

Describes the characteristics of the American black from the standpoint of the physical anthropologist. It was found that, in general, the head of the American black is about 2 millimeters narrower than the head of the white. Consonant with this form, the elevation of the black head is lower by about 5 millimeters. Other anthropometric characters are as follows: 1) Cranial capacity less; 2) Hair line lower on forehead; 3) Interpupillary Distance greater; 4) Nose Height less; 5) Bridge of nose lower; 6) Nose broader; torso shorter; arm longer; 7) Progmathism greater; 8) Lips thicker; External ear shorter; 9) Chest shallower; Pelvis narrower and smaller; and 10) Leg longer; weight heavier; stature shorter. These characters are the "Condition in the American Black as compared with Old American Whites or mixed Europeans." Concludes with the observation that "The American Negro represents an amalgam into which had entered the genes of African Negroes, whites of all nations and social classes, and American Indians, and that as far as his physical characters are concerned the American Negro represents the successful blending of these three principal elements into the unique biological type which he is."

320. Moody, V. Alton. "Slavery on Louisiana Sugar Plantations," Louisiana Historical Quarterly 7 (1924):191-301.

The text is divided into seven parts, the fifth of which
deals with "the necessities of life." Under this
heading the author discusses "housing, food and water,
clothing, and care of the sick and helpless."
Segregation of sick slaves appears to have been one of
the only means of preventive health care. In 1806, the
Territory of Orleans passed an act which established a
code of conduct for the treatment of sick slaves.
Owners were obligated to feed and maintain even those
slaves with incurable diseases. Because of this
requirement and the economic benefits involved in
keeping slaves healthy, most planters paid a flat fee
for a poorly trained and poorly equipped physician to
make periodic rounds. Points out that black females
often acted as medical assistants to the physicians and
with some training, "rendered services to the Negroes
almost equal to that rendered the whites." Observes
that owners took pains to see that pregnant slaves and
slaves who had recently given birth were not overworked.
Newborns were kept in the master's house and were cared
for by the owner's family and (periodically) by the
mother of the child.

321. Moseley, John E. "Cancer and the Negro," Crisis 56 (5)
(May 1949):138-139, 156.

Discusses the pecularities about cancer as it affects
blacks. The first pecularity is the relative immunity
of blacks of skin cancer. "The prevalence of skin
cancer in white males is reported to be about ten times
as great as in Negro males, and in white females about
six times as great in Negro females." Another unusual
feature of cancer in blacks is the high rate of uterus
cancer in black females. Cancer is 63 percent higher
among black females than among white females. The
disease is also found at an earlier age in black women
than in white women. Notes that the high incidences of
cancer among black women may be the result of injuries
sustained in childbirth. Concludes that blacks would
have a greater chance of living if cancer was detected
in a curable stage. In order for this earlier detection
to occur, blacks must be educated about cancer and its
warning signs. In addition to educating blacks,
recommends the need for more advanced training
opportunities for black physicians and the need to make
medical facilities more accessible to blacks.

322. Mountin, Joseph W. "The Appraisal of Programs for
Medical and Hospital Care in Small Towns and Rural Areas," In
National Conference of Catholic Charities, Proceedings of the
Twenty-Sixth Meeting...Chicago, Illinois, November 17 to 20,
1940 (Washington, DC: The Conference, 1941): 140-152.

Discusses the problems of providing adequate medical and
hospital care for residents of rural areas, particularly
for blacks who have very small incomes. Uses data from
the National Health Survey to show rural medical needs
and the difference between rural and urban areas in

amount of physicians' services, hospital care, and
nursing care received by sick persons.

323. Mudge, Gertrude G. "A Comparative Study of Italian,
Polish, and Negro Dietaries," Journal of the American
Dietetic Association 1 (1925/1926):166-173.

Three years ago the Social Service Section of the
American Dietetic Association initiated a series of
studies of the dietary habits of different nationalities
in several large cities in the U.S. A total of 107
families were studied (36 Polish, 38 Italians and 44
blacks). The study examined amount spent per person for
food items of various costs, amount spent total per
month, and at the percent of calories, protein, calcium,
phosphorous and iron the groups averaged. It appears
that blacks on average brought lower cost food items
compared to Pols and Italians and that blacks
comparatively received lower percentages of recommended
amounts of calories, protein, calcium, phosphorous and
iron than the other two groups. Concludes that with
limited incomes, the appropriate diet is difficult,
however, dietary education can help to improve the
current intake.

324. Mullowney, John J. "The Weakest Link." Journal of
Medical Education 4 (1929): 205-207.

The question examined is whether or not there are any
communitites in the country that adequately provide for
the education, sanitation and the public health of
blacks. There are only two black medical schools
recognized by the American Medical Association
graduating only some 100 black physicians a year.

325. Mullowney, John J. "The Effect of the Depression on
Medical Students of the Negro Group and on Internships
Available." Journal of Medical Education 10 (1935):218-225.

Compares conditions in 1929 with conditions in 1934 in
black medical colleges and hospitals. The results show:
there has been a marked decrease in the number of blacks
in the northern and eastern medical schools; black
hospitals are improving and increasing in number,
however, two had lost recognition, in the period
1929-1933, inclusive; and several of the southern states
have no recognized hospitals or physicians and this is
where the larger population of blacks are located.

326. Murray, Florence. "Hospitals," The Negro Handbook
(February 1, 1942): 152.

Notes that 5,838 new beds had been installed for the
care of "colored patients in hospitals throughout the
south." The new beds were made available through
grants-in-aid programs. A total of 3,486 beds or 59.7
percent were provided for the insane, 1,464 or 25.2
percent were provided in tuberculosis sanitaria and
other specialized hospitals. One of the largest

hospitals erected for blacks at that time was the Homer
G. Phillips Municipal Hospital in St. Louis. This
facility had a capacity of 685 beds. Another municipal
hospital for blacks was the Norfolk Community Hospital
with a capacity of 54 beds. In 1941, $700,000 was
granted to Freedmen's Hospital at Washington, D.C. to
build a tuberculosis annex for "colored" patients. Also
built in 1941 was the Infantile Paralysis Center at
Tuskegee Institute. It was the first of its kind for
"exclusive use by Negroes in the United States." The
center provided treatment for children and adults
affected with poliomyelitis or handicapped as a result
of the disease. It also provided valuable training for
"colored" doctors, physical therapists, and nurses in
the treatment of poliomyelitis.

327. Murray, Florence. "National Negro Health Movement,"
The Negro Handbook (July 1944): 194.

Describes the activities which occurred during the
annual National Negro Health Week. However, unlike the
aforementioned week, the health movement was year round.
The National Negro Health Movement solicited support
from various health organizations to help educate blacks
in the prevention of diseases prevalent to them. This
movement was established by Booker T. Washington. The
projects undertaken during the health week included
cleaning up homes, insect control activities, "outhouse"
improvements and clinical treatment to name a few.

328. Murray, Florence. "Some Facts and Figures on
Hospitals," The Negro Handbook (February 1942): 153.

Points out the many improvements and building of
designated hospitals for the care of black patients.
The instrumental force behind the improvements was the
National Hospital Association. As of 1942, "there were
110 Negro hospitals throughout the U.S. with more than
10,000 beds specifically to treat Negroes." More than
70 percent of the hospitals were privately owned.

329. Mustard, H. S. and Waring, J. I. "Heights and Weights
of Colored School Children," American Journal of Public
Health 16 (Fall 1926):1017-1021.

Investigations show that the colored race has a growth
cycle which differs in many respects from that of the
white. The purpose of the study was to determine the
proper way to administer a health program for both
blacks and whites. Studies show that although among
adults there is a tendency for colored and white to have
about the same height. The weight of colored males was
shown to be uniformly above the weight of white males.

330. Myers, Arthur. "Tuberculosis Among Negroes." Hygiene
(1932): 586-587.

The black race was said to be free from tuberculosis
before the days of the European and Arabian traders and

conquers of Africa. Before the Civil War blacks in the
United States had good living conditions. However,
after the Civil War blacks were dying from tuberculosis
at the same rate as whites. This was due to the poor
living conditions of blacks after the war.

331. Myers, Beatrice A. and Reid, Ira A. "The Toll of
Tuberculosis Among Negroes in New Jersey," Opportunity 10 (9)
(September 1932): 279-282.

The astounding neglect of the health of blacks in the
State of New Jersey is discussed. In New Jersey during
1930, 264 blacks died from tuberculosis for each 100,000
in the population, while 58 whites per 100,000 died from
this disease. The black population of New Jersey was
dying 4.6 times higher from tuberculosis as the white
population. Only three southern states had black
tuberculosis death rates higher than that in New Jersey
in 1927. In 1930 the white tuberculosis death rate was
45.2 percent lower than in 1920. The rate for blacks in
1930, however, was only 7.9 percent lower than in 1920.
Discusses the significance of these numbers by an
examination of specific death rates by age. Points out
studies that showed that very little work was being done
in many parts of the state of New Jersey and that no
plan had been introduced to solve the problem.

332. Myers, H. J. and Leon, Y. "Color Denial in the Negro:
A Preliminary Report," Psychiatry 11 (1) (February 1948):
39-46.

Discusses the frequency of concern with color in black
psychotics and the color notion both in the white and
black communities. The existence of a caste system and
of stereotyped notions about blacks have been indicated.
These notions affect the black community and white
standards and white ideals are often taken as desirable
goals. Whiteness represents full participation in
American democratic society and "superior advantage,
achievement, progress and power all of which have great
significance for survival." The use of skin lighteners
and hair straighteners are the given examples in the
expression of the blacks dreams and phantasies. The
psychosis often includes elements which reflect a need
to solve the problem of color and the difficulties in
living associated with being black.

333. Nathan, A. and Altschul, A. "Diabetes in Harlem
Hospital Outpatient Department in New York," Journal of the
American Medical Association 119 (May 1942): 248-253.

The authors contribute small pieces of their current
work which is pertinent to the dietetic field in some
way, shape or form. Finds that the mortality rate for
female black diabetic patients has increased 75 percent
in seven years, and 26 percent for female white patients
over the same period and that the onset of the diabetes
in the black patient is much earlier than in the white
patient. Heredity and familial incidence are factors in

etiology but obesity is predominate in both white and black patients and diet may be a factor in the variance of mortality rates. Therefore, diet of the black diabetic should be a focal point in treatment.

334. Nathan, Winfred B. "Health Education in Negro Public Schools," Journal of Negro Education 6 (1937): 523-530.

Before addressing the main topic of the article, the author briefly reviews the health status of blacks, emphasizing the problems of tuberculosis and infant mortality. He then discusses the family life of the typical black school-age youngster, noting that we must understand the background of black youngsters if we are to understand what public schools can and cannot do to improve black health. Points out that an effective program must influence home life. In examining the health programs of Southern states, the author finds these programs to be well-conceived but poorly implemented. Argues that black schools are woefully underfunded and poorly equipped. The schools themselves are often unsanitary, thus it is hardly surprising that there is an inadequate health education program. Reports the findings of a study of 18 black secondary schools in Georgia and argues that public schools must share the responsibility for the improvement of black's social environment.

335. National Negro Health Association, "Activities for National Negro Health Week: March 31-April 7, 1940," National Negro Health Week 26 (1940): 9-14.

The first week of April was recognized as National Negro Health Week. A variety of seminars, lectures, and preventive medicine was offered. The activities for the 26th observance included various community health day, home health day, etc. Doctors examined blacks, expressing the importance of a balanced daily diet and social hygiene. The doctors explained that tuberculosis, syphilis, cancer, and organic diseases were the chief causes of disability and death.

336. "National Negro Health Week," American Journal of Public Health 12 (Summer 1922):528.

A brief discussion of the year's Negro Health Week conducted by the Tuskegee Institute. The purpose of the week was to reduce morbidity and mortality among blacks by educational methods, with particular emphasis on tuberculosis, infant mortality and venereal diseases.

337. "Negro Doctors to Serve in Veterans' Hospitals." National Negro Health News 14 (2) (1946): 2.

Dr. Paul R. Hawley, Veteran's Administration medical director, reports that the way has been cleared for appointment of black doctors in veteran's hospitals. Local customs are to be the ruling factor in making the appointments. He is considering plans to set up all black units in a number of hospitals with black patients to be attended by black doctors and nurses.

338. "Negro Insurance Association Adopts Social Hygiene Resolution," Journal of Social Hygiene 32 (7) (October 1946): 335-336.

The annual conference of the Negro United Insurance Association, held in the Harlem District of New York City on July 9-12, adopted its resolution. The resolution was presented by the Harlem Council on Social Hygiene, Incorporated, and was unanimously adopted by the 61 black insurance agencies and the ten regional Associations comprising the United Negro Insurance Association. "Because the venereal disease problem is a major health hazard to the American Negro; and because we are vitally interested in seeing this menance eradicated, be it therefore resolved that the United Negro Insurance Association in convention assembled, New York City, July 9-12 endorses local and national social hygiene programs and actively support them in their home communities." During the conference, 1,500 pieces of literature and 5,000 educational match books were distributed to the delegates.

339. "Negro Medical Center Planned at Provident Hospital, Chicago," National Negro Health News (January - March, 1946): 3.

Noted physicians are planning to establish Provident Hospital as a national center for black medical training and research. The team of Scribner and Fitz-Hugh will provide supplementary activities of the hospital and training schools. Provident Hospital is "already one of the outstanding Negro institutions in the country." Chicago's four major medical schools would be the support team for the medical facility.

340. "Negroes and Group Health," New Republic 114 (April 22, 1946):566.

Points out that blacks will for the first time be included in the Group Health Association. This program extends comprehensive, high-quality medical care and hospital protection to 3,100 federal employees and their families. By a vote of 1,133 to 528, the members of the Association agreed to accept blacks into the plan. The motion regarding their inclusion contained the provision that no racial discrimination would be made with regard either to individual or to group admissions. It is believed that this is the first provision of its kind. This proposal was rejected two years earlier because of the fear that blacks were bad physical risks. Medical evidence was cited, however, to prove that susceptibility to disease is an economic rather than a racial factor.

341. "Negroes Hard Hit by Tuberculosis," American Journal of Public Health, 24 (February 1934):154.

Tuberculosis is the cause of death among blacks in a far
greater percentage than among whites. Nearly one-fourth
of all deaths from tuberculosis in Illinois are among
blacks and other colored races, although they make up
less than one-twentieth of the population. Mortality
from tuberculosis among blacks in Illinois is six times
greater than among whites. The progress toward
eradicating tuberculosis in Illinois has been much less
among blacks than among whites. Blacks have had a
nineteen percent decline, whereas whites enjoy a
forty-five percent reduction. Only heart impairment
causes greater mortality rates among blacks. The
rigorous Illinois climate was given as a factor in the
alarming tuberculosis death rates.

342.   "Negroes Help Themselves," American Journal of Public
Health 39 (August 1949):1026.

Discusses a 1947-48 pilot health program in Webster
Parish, Louisiana. Of the population of 35,000, nearly
half were blacks. Ninety-two percent of the 3,500
blacks school children were given medical examinations.
Eighty-three percent required treatment. Forty percent
of the children had throat defects, thirty percent,
nutrition defects, and twenty percent, defects of the
teeth. Followup treatment was given to these children
during the school year. The health program consisted of
100 percent dental, eye, and chest x-ray examinations,
nutrition service through school cafeterias, and
development of a preschool health service.

343.   "Negro Medical Schools." Journal of Medical Education
4 (1929):320.

At the thirty-ninth annual meeting of the Association of
American Medical Colleges a resolution was presented by
Dr. E. P. Lyon, dean of the University of Minnesota
Medical School, and it was unamiously accepted. The
resolution stated that better facilities for the
education of black physicians and nurses were needed;
that the attention of philanthropic citizens and
foundations be directed to the opportunities afforded in
the field of black medical education; and that attention
be called to the excellent work being done against odds
at the Howard University Medical School and the Meharry
Medical School, and to the needs of these institutions
for buildings, hospital facilities, equipment and
endowment.

344.   "Negro Participation in the American Red Cross
Program." National Negro Health News 14 (3) (1946): 11-13.

Increasing black participation and leadership in the
nutrition, home nursing, first aid, water safety and
accident prevention program of the American Red Cross
was pointed out by Red Cross Chairman Basil O'Connor in
announcing the cooperation of the organization with the
32nd observance of National Negro Health Week, Narch 31
- April 7, 1946. One of the principle aims of the Red

Cross is to raise the health standards of the total population.

345. "Negro Students in Medical Schools." Journal of Medical Education   23 (1948):   270-271.

A summary of black medical freshmen students as reported by the medical schools of the United States at a total of 162. Of that number, 70 are enrolled in Howard University School of Medicine and 66 were enrolled in 22 other medical schools with not more than 2 at any one of these schools. The number enrolled is 3 per cent of the total freshmen medical enrollment.

346. "New Jersey Hospitals Work Toward Eliminating Racial Discrimination." The Modern Hospital, February, 1950. Cited in National Negro Health News 18 (2) (1950): 21.

New Jersey hospitals were credited with progress toward the elimination of racial discrimination in a report issued last month by the State Department of Education in cooperation with the New Jersey Hospital Association. The report summarized the findings of a survey covering admission and placement practices in 85 voluntary hospitals located in 21 counties throughout the state. Some discriminatory policies exist in hospitals, it was reported, but "the trend seems to be toward non-discrimination where hospitals are concerned." Practices in a number of hospitals and nursing schools were liberalized during the period covered by the survey.

347. Nichols, Franklin O. "Some Public Health Problems of the Negro," Journal of Social Hygiene 8 (3) (July 1922): 281-285.

Presents data indicative of the prevalence of diseases resulting in morbidity and mortality and suggests that the church organization be included in the programs designed to reduce and prevent deaths. Finds no valid data dealing with black morbidity and mortality, but that the important diseases affecting blacks are tuberculosis, the various infantile diseases, pellagra and venereal disease (compiled by some of the leading insurance companies). According to Metropolitan Life Insurance Company, tuberculosis is exacting a toll on about eleven times as many black boys and about eight times as many young black girls as whites. After the age of 35, there is not much difference in the effect of the diseases in the two races. The average death rate of black babies is approximately 200 per 1000 births. Notes that gonorrhea and syphilis are responsible for insanity, paralysis, sterility, organic heart trouble, locomotor ataxia and other pathological conditions. Advocates that the church cooperate in eliminating diseases by educating the black community to the overindulgence of appetites; by informing members of the importance of fresh air, wholesome food, and a balanced diet in addition to persuading members to have a

physical examination once a year; and by stressing the
need for a monagamous home in our racial life. Special
attention to the psychology of children and adolescence
is important in molding the character and developing the
elements of a personality - a task for the church in
educating the family.

348. Nichols, Franklin O. "Social Hygiene and the Negro,"
Journal of Social Hygiene 15 (7) (October 1929): 408-413.

Social hygiene work with the American black has been
extended to include the preparation of black youth for
marriage and parenthood. Views the difficult and
hazardous history of blacks due to the institution of
slavery as underlying cause for the development and
widespread diseases among the black race. The
institution of slavery required no regulation of sexual
activity, no tradition of family and no knowledge of the
importance of sex and reproduction in individual and
racial health. In addition to this, the race faced
problems of adjusting itself to a complicated social and
economic environment with a heritage of poverty,
illiteracy, a lack of education and health
opportunities, and disenfranchisement stemming from
interracial relations. All of these factors affect the
stability and vitality of family life. Thus, is was
inevitable that the race would develop problems of
common-law marriages, unstable families, illigetimacy
and a prevalence of venereal disease. After 60 years of
struggle for improvement, the black race revealed a
tremendous racial capacity for adjustment which
demonstrates the vitality of the race. The social
hygiene program has included plans for assisting black
families in preparing their youth for the
responsibilities and realities of marriage. Scientific
lectures have incorporated biological, psychological,
sociological, physiological and ethical knowledge into
their curriculum. Finally, black high schools are
beginning to be reached in the promotion of this work,
and are considering English and the social sciences as
primary value courses for cultivating attitudes on
behalf of the student with reference to the problems of
marriage and child rearing.

349. Nichols, Franklin O. "Social Hygiene in Racial
Problems-The Negro," Journal of Social Hygiene 28 (8)
(November 1932): 446-451.

Points out that the American Social Hygiene Association
two main objectives are: (1) to promote sex hygiene in
educational institutions for blacks, and (2) to continue
an intensive campaign against syphilis and gonorrhea.
Black education leaders had become discouraged in their
efforts to meet the sex educational needs of students
and welcomed the opportunity to cooperate in raising the
subject of sex and reproduction to a level of
educational dignity. This includes black leadership
concerns with the improvement of the family as a
significant element in racial progress and health. This

effort resulted in the elimination of undesirable
approaches to this subject and cleared the way for the
inclusion of sex educational subject matter in courses
in physiology and hygiene, psychology, sociology,
biology, education, and home economics as a part of the
regular curriculum in schools and colleges for blacks.
The three public health conditions which threatens the
health of blacks are tuberculosis, syphilis, and
conditions affecting childhood and infancy. Much work
has been done over the past ten years through lectures,
movie films and literature on syphilis and gonorrhea.
But, due to limited funds and insufficient personnel,
the greatest proportion of the black masses have not
been reached. The spread of venereal disease among
blacks is complicated by environmental factors such as
the high cost of medical treatment, and social and
economic conditions. Concludes that in the effort to
reduce and control venereal disease among blacks, a
steady pressure is being applied for the elimination of
quacks and charlatans who exploit blacks and to get
druggists to cooperate to eliminate damaging "over the
counter" prescriptions for venereal diseases.

350. Niles, George M.   "Afro-American Therapeutics," New
Orleans Medical and Surgical Journal 78 (April 1926):747-749.

Addresses the duty of white physicians to take care of
the "hybrid" Afro-American and discusses differences
between the Afro-American and the Caucasian. Blacks
require less morphine than the Caucasian to take care of
pain, rarely suffers from insomnia or psychiatric
problems, and have much thicker skin than the Caucasian.
Concludes with a discussion that blacks are much more
receptive to psychotherapy and blacks tend to cooperate
fully with the therapist whereas the Caucasian displays
a "show-me" attitude. Psychotherapy combined with
medicinal measures yield highly superior results for the
primitively-developed mentalities of Afro-Americans.

351. Olsen, Edwin.   "Social Aspects of Slave Life in New
York," The Journal of Negro History 26 (January 1941): 66-77.

Focuses on small scale slaveholding in the state of New
York ranging on the average of holding of 2.4 blacks per
every white owner. The main purpose of slaveholding was
to obtain dividends in the form of labor services.
Provides vivid descriptions of slave life ranging from
mistreatment by the owners to food, clothing, housing,
and health care to death. Ill or injured slaves were
cared for to prevent financial loss which occurred if an
ill slave of working age died or became incapacitated
permanently. According to the documents of the Lloyd
Family, in 1730, the family physician, Dr. George
Murison, prescribed many forms of treatment for "a Gouty
Rumatic Disorder," such as purging, powders, diet
drinks, bloodletting and applications of ointments.
Suggests that yellow fever affected blacks the least.
When the disease swept New York City in 1805, 1819, 1822
and 1823 killing hundreds of whites, deaths among blacks

were negligible. Thought to be immune, blacks proved
valuable in attending to the stricken and burying the
dead. Most of the whites fled from Manhattan Island
with the arrival of the disease.

352. "One Part of the Jig-saw Puzzle." Abstract from an
Editorial in The Informer, June, 1935, Bulletin of the Urban
League of Pittsburgh. Cited in National Negro Health News 3
(2) (1935): 12-13.

Sponsored by a Citizen's Committee, the Social Study of
Pittsburgh and Allegheny County undertook the job of
taking apart, carefully examining, evaluating, and
placing together again a giant jig-saw puzzle - the
social work structure of the community. One of the
first of the reports released by the Committee was "The
Organized Care of the Sick" prepared by Dr. Gertrude
Sturges. The report discusses hospital care,
out-patient service, convalescent care, etc., with a
special section devoted to "The Medical Care of the
Negro." It discusses their opportunities for medical
education and training and the chief problems.

353. Oppenheim, A. "Health Education in Action," American
Journal of Public Health 33 (November 1943):1339-1342.

This article, written by the Director of the Bienville
Parish Health Unit in Arcadia, Louisiana, focuses on a
before and after project. Before 1942, Roberson, a
typical rural black settlement in Bienville Parish, had
barely utilized the services of the county health unit.
Of the 55 families that made up this community, several
had brought infants and youngsters to child health
conferences; some had received the typhoid vaccine,
while a few others had undergone treatment for syphilis.
This constituted the total contact with the health unit.
One year later, the community had its own health clinic
operated by volunteers from all of the families. Points
out how education of the community can make a
difference.

354. Ornstein, George. "The Leading Cause of Death Among
Negroes: Tuberculosis," Journal of Negro Education 6 (1937):
303-313.

In 1934, tuberculosis along with pneumonia accounted for
over 30 percent of total deaths among the black
population in the City of New York. Although initial
infections closely resemble that in the white race,
subsequent infections are much more severe and fatal.
Researchers have attempted to account for these
differences using physical, anatomical, and
environmental factors. Early records from the health
office in Charleston, South Carolina reveal that blacks
respond much better than whites to the disease when it
first emerges. However, after 1865 these results
changed drastically and blacks began to endure much
higher mortality rates. This date coincides with the
emancipation of blacks at which time they were left to

their own resources, and faced the worst environmental
and economic problems of any race. Most researchers
have concluded that disparities in mortality reflect
differences in economic conditions. Most blacks
inflicted with the disease were already suffering from
numerous other infectious diseases associated with poor
diets, insanitary living quarters, and poor social
hygiene. Clinicians in many municipalities have found
similarities in the course of infection in many whites
who suffer from similar environmental conditions.

355.   "Orthopedic Unit Certifies First Negro Surgeon."
National Negro Health News 16 (3) (1949): 24.

The American Board of Orthopedic Surgery certified Dr.
J. Robert Gladden, a Washington, D.C. physician, the
first black to qualify in this specialty. Dr. Gladden
is on the orthopedic staffs of the Howard University
School of Medicine and Freedmen's Hospital. A graduate
of Long Island University and Meharry Medical College,
he served his internship at Provident Hospital,
Baltimore. He has written several articles on diseases
of the bones and joints and is the first resident in
orthopedic surgery at Freedmen's Hospital.

356.   Osborne, Estelle Massey. "Status and Contribution of
the Negro Nurse," The Journal of Negro Education 18 (Summer
1949):364-369.

With the assertion that "professional relations in
nursing are so interwoven with race relations that it is
imperative for Negro nurses to move on both fronts
simultaneously," the author outlines the status of black
nurses along three sets of circumstances: World War II,
Critical Studies of the Nursing Profession and the
National Shortage of Nurses. Shortages in nursing
caused by World War II led many institutions to open
doors to qualified black nursing students. Between 1941
and 1949, 325 additional schools opened doors to blacks
for training. Following the war, the National Nursing
Council, solidified by the war, was in a position to
evaluate the progress and problems of the nursing
profession. These evaluations led to recommendations
that 'minority groups' be included in future plans for
the profession. Trends toward the extension of health
services to a larger part of the population than before
are creating an increasing demand for nurses. In the
interest of supplying this demand, the nursing
profession is broadening its "recruiting appeal" to
include black youths in the opportunities which now
exist in nursing. In conclusion, points out that the
nursing profession has surpassed other professions in
integration of its work force.

357.   Oxley, Lawrence A. "North Carolina and Her Crippled
Negro Children," Southern Workman 60 (February 1931): 74-78.

The author explains that care for cripples is usually
limited to the orthopedic defects of childhood and that

North Carolina has managed to grasp opportunities that
promote hygiene. The North Carolina Orthopedic Hospital
at Gastonia offers services to indigent crippled
children under 16 at no cost. When the author visited
the hospital, she wondered why no black children were
present, and only a small percent of white children were
actually admitted. This was due to small amounts of
funding. Black children, however, received limited
treatment at other clinics elsewhere. In 1926, Mr. B.
N. Duke gave a gift of $15,000 to erect a building at
the hospital site, for the hospitalization of crippled
black children. This gesture received a favorable
response from many of the state's citizens.

358. Parran, Thomas. "A General Introductory Statement to
the Problems of the Health Status and Health Education of
Negroes," Journal of Negro Education 6 (1937): 263-267.

Blacks have suffered unusual problems in regard to
specific diseases. These diseases have resulted in
increased incidences of illnesses and mortality among
blacks in comparisons to whites. Such diseases as
cancer, mental insanity, infant and maternal mortality,
tuberculosis and syphilis has caused increased detriment
to black health status. An already poor health status
is in jeopardy of becoming worse. However, there are
means through which the health status of blacks can be
improved. By educating the black to utilize
satisfactory dietary methods and improving sanitation in
his living quarters, unnecessary sickness and premature
death may be prevented. The preservation of black
health status is contingent on adequate health
education. Viruses associated with specific diseases
are manifested only in susceptable host organisms.
Blacks must utilize health education to retard the
colonization of parasites and other diseases.

359. Parran, Thomas. "Public Health - The Base of
Progress," Opportunity 23 (4) (Fall 1945): 195-197.

Notes that poverty, ignorance, and lack of medical care
form the base upon which ill health builds in all
communities and among all races. Emphasizes that too
many inequalities exist in society in that blacks
constitute 10 percent of our population, but they bear
from three to six times their proportional burden of ill
health and premature death. Discusses numerous other
racial inequities that occur and views the following
requirements as basic for the operation of a democratic
society: full employment, with a continuing rise in
income and standard of living; equal opportunity for
education; and equal opportunity for health. Stresses
that health is a problem of the whole nation and that
one of the first steps to be taken to solve it is for
the people themselves to study their health problems and
determine their needs. Although the specific needs of
communities and population groups vary in kind and in
quantity, the author believes that the major health
requirements throughout the country are for better

facilities and more trained personnel. Concludes with a
brief examination of recent medical developments such as
penicillin and treatment facilities.

360. Parris, G. "American College of Surgeons Admits Negro
Candidates," Opportunity 25 (1) (January 1947): 29.

The American College of Surgeons prior to 1947 had
restricted membership for blacks. Points out the eight
black candidates who were sent notices to report for
initiation ceremonies during the annual clinical
congress in Cleveland. Dr. Malcolm T. MacEachern,
associate director of the college, also announced that
four other blacks had been admitted as fellows in
November 1945. During that year, the society did not
hold a congress and the candidates were notified by mail
of their acceptance in the society. Those surgeons
notified included doctors from New York, New Jersey, and
Philadelphia. Candidates for fellowships had to be
graduates of an acceptable medical school, with three
years of hospital experience. In addition, they must
have devoted seven years to special training and must
submit 100 care records of major surgical work.

361. Paullin, J. E., Davison, H. M. and Wood, R. W.
"Incidence of Syphilitic Infection Among Negroes in the
South," Boston Medical and Scientific Journal 197 (September
1927):345-350.

A report of a study made in the early 1920s and
considers the influence of syphilis in causing various
physical and mental disabilities, and discusses the
methods, both effective and ineffective, which were
currently being used to combat the disease.

362. Pearl, Raymond. "Biological Factors in Negro
Mortality," Human Biology 2 (May 1929): 229-249.

Argues that external biological differences between the
black and whites races are reflected internally as well.
Blacks react differently to diseases than whites in a
great many ways, including incidence, organical, and
etc. In fact, researchers felt that the racial
differences discovered in pathology were so great, that
it seemed reasonable to use the findings to help plan
health programs for blacks. In some areas, blacks
appear to enjoy a greater biological fitness than their
counterpart, while in other respects, blacks are
distinctly less adapted to the general environment in
which they must live.

363. Perrott, George and Holland, Dorothy. "The Need for
Current Data on Illnesses Among Negroes," Journal of Negro
Education 6 (1937): 350-362.

For any public health program to be effective, there
must be well documented records pertaining to the rate
of illnesses and mortality in each race. The data would
allow researchers to examine the essential differences

in characteristics of the mortality rate in the white
and black populations. Because such data would provide
the initial evidence of susceptability to certain
diseases and illnesses, researchers would be able to
address these disparities long before any significant
death toll is allowed to accumulate. Without such data,
variation in regard to age, sex, urbanization and
economic status of morbidity characteristics among
blacks cannot be defined. As a result, the ability to
isolate the variable contributing to the fatality rates
would become impossible to isolate.

364. Pevaroff, H. H. and Hindman, S. M. "The Dick Test in
White and Negro Children," American Journal of Hygiene 19
(May 1934):749-752.

The Dick test, concerning medical conditions resulting
from malnutrition and named after its developer Dr.
George Frederick Dick (1881-1967), was conducted among
black children who lived in overcrowded sections of
Cleveland, Ohio in the 1920s and early 1930s.

365. Phillips, L. D. "Comparative Incidence of
Tuberculosis," Delaware State Medical Journal 10 (August
1938):170-172.

Investigates whether there was a specifically racial
aspect to tuberculosis, or whether it was strictly a
disease of poverty caused by poor nutrition and hygiene.
Compares incidence of tuberculosis occurring among the
white and the black populations in the state of
Delaware.

366. "Physical Check-Up During National Health Week,"
National Negro Health News 3 (July - September 1949): 9.

In Pemiscot and Dunklin Counties, Missouri, 2,044 rural
black school children were given free physical
examinations. The examinations were sponsored by the
Home Economics Extension County Council and the Negro
Health Advisory Committee. This was the first clinic of
its kind to be held on a county-wide basis in Missouri.

367. Pipkin, A. C. and Pipkin, S. B. "Ear Pits and Albinism
in a Negro Family," The Journal of Heredity 43 (1943):
240-242.

Discusses a black family in which both albinism and ear
pits were transmitted from the mother. Three of her
five children inherited both traits, one son inherited
albinism only, and one son inherited neither
abnormality. Focuses on the genetic possibilities of
such an unusual occurrence. Photographs of the family
are provided with close-ups of the ears (showing the
presence or absence of ear pits).

368. Pizzolato, P. "Leukemia in the Negro," Journal of the
National Medical Association 41 (September 1949): 214-219.

Not many studies have been published on the incidence and frequency of leukemia in blacks. From a study of 85 patients during the years 1937 to 1947, it seemed that the incidence of leukemia was less in blacks at a large southern center. Irrespective of treatment, shorter life span of patients with leukemia were found as a result of the disease. Sicklemia was also found in some of the patients.

369. Poindexter, Hildrus A. "Handicaps in the Normal Growth and Development of Rural Negro Children," American Journal of Public Health 28 (September 1938):1048-52.

The problem of the handicapped rural black is becoming increasingly serious. He is becoming more and more recognized as a reservoir for certain illnesses, such as venereal disease and malaria. The rural black is handicapped not only because he harbors certain microorganisms that are associated with his environment, but by lack of socio-intellectual facilities and opportunities. Non-infectious malnutrition is one disease of the rural black. It is characterized by flabby muscles, poor posture and eyesight, pellagric conditions of the skin, and dental caries. Syphilis is a second common illness. Because of promiscuity, this disease is quickly spreading throughout the black community. Thirdly, malaria is prevalent among southern blacks. It is 4.2 to 6 times more common in blacks than in whites. Lastly, hookworm infestation is costly to black health. Incidence among black children between nine and fourteen years of age may be as high as twenty percent. Chief factors responsible for these problems include ignorance, poverty, and inadequate social agencies.

370. Poindexter, H. A. "Special Health Problems of Negroes in Rural Areas," Journal of Negro Education 6 (1937):399-412.

This study is a summary of data drawn from U.S. Census reports, records from the U.S. Department of Education, and various annual reports and records from several southern states. Concludes that "improper diet, insanitary [sic] environment, and ignorance of personal hygiene and of the hazard of local customs and occupations" were the bases of health problems faced by rural blacks in the 1930s. Improper diet was the result of planting vegetables in one season only and not canning vegetables for the other times of the year. Malaria and hookworm were the consequences of unsanitary living conditions. Hookworm infestation could be reduced by the use of "sanitary privies" to prevent "soil pollution by human excretion." Ignorance of personal hygiene especially manifested itself in the form of syphilis. Programs of sex education "graded for age, sex, and intelligency" were necessary to reduce the rate of venereal diseases. The author charges the health departments of southern states to accept blacks as citizens and cease discrimination in disease prevention. Also urges state boards of education and

public school teachers to take more of a role in
educating blacks on how to prevent disease.

371. Porter, William P. and Walker, Harry. "Hyperthyroidism
in the Negro," Annals of Internal Medicine 11 (1937-38):
618-625.

In this case study of hyperthyroidism in blacks, it is
revealed that the malady is relatively common to blacks.
The disease manifests itself clinically as typical
Graves' disease and is accompanied by a diffuse
hyperplasia of the thyroid gland. The cutaneous changes
are of peculiar interest and of real diagnostic
importance. The cardiovascular apparatus of the black
patient suffers greatly from the effects of
hyperthyroidism largely because of delay in seeking
adequate treatment. Some factors other than primary
codine deficiency or the stress of urban life must be
found to explain adequately the pathogenesis of
expohthalmic goiter.

372. "Post War Health Program in West Virginia," The Negro
History Bulletin 8 (Summer 1944-1945):40-42.

Focuses on the importance of the health of all citizens
of the United States. Education has been proclaimed as
the need of a large part of our citizenry. To help with
this education, West Virginia has built the outstanding
Health Building at the West Virginia State College. It
is well equipped with everything required by the staff
of physical directors, doctors, and nurses employed to
parallel the development of the body along with that of
the mind. This recently completed building, costing
about one-half a million, is the pride of the campus.

373. "Postgraduate Training of Negro Physicians in the
Clinical Management and Public Health Control of Syphilis,"
Journal of Social Hygiene 23 (8) (November 1937): 454.

An announcement was made by the United States Public
Health Service to state health officials and other
interested parties, that the District of Columbia Health
Department in arrangement with the Howard University
Medical School formed the organization of a special
course of postgraduate training of black physicians in
the clinical managment and public health control of
syphilis and gonorrhea. The planned course of
instruction would extend over a period of three months
and would be repeated for successive periods during the
following year beginning September 1, 1937. There would
be fifteen (15) members per class with a new class to be
registered every three months. Instructions would
provide lectures and clinical and laboratory
demonstrations for training in the clinical management
of syphilis and gonorrhea. Trainees would be selected
by the State health officers. Traveling expenses and
other allowances would be charged against the allotment
made to the respective States for training and reserve
personnel for the fiscal year 1937-1938. Candidate

preference would be given to well-trained young black physicians who were expected to participate in local and state syphilis control program in the capacity of venereal disease control officers, consultants and cooperating clinicians with health departments.

374. "Premedical Education for Negroes." Journal of Medical Education 4 (1929):110-112.

Discusses issue of quality premedical education for blacks. Several black colleges offer premedical courses proposing to prepare men in two years to enter medical college. Questions the fairness of these institutions to the men who may be attracted by such offers, if after pursuing two years, they cannot enter a recognized medical college.

375. Puffer, Ruth Rice. "Measurement of Error of Death Rates in the Colored Race," American Journal of Public Health 27 (June 1937):603-8.

Notes that fifty-eight percent of the colored population in the United States are living in twelve states in the South. In 1933, the average urban death rate in these areas was 20.5 percent, or sixty-one percent higher than the rural death rate of 12.7. Points out that the accuracy of the death rates from specific causes depends on many factors. First, the size of the rates will depend upon the completeness of the registration. Second, the accuracy of the death rates will depend on the quality of certification of causes of death and the amount of variation in the type of certification. The attendance at death and the certification of causes of death by physicians are essential.

376. "Race Prejudice in Municipal Hospitals," Editorial, Opportunity, (August 1941): 10.

An investigation of race prejudice in the Lincoln Hospital was conducted by a committee of the City Council of the City of New York. The Jewish physicians on the staff of the hospital were never promoted to high ranking staff positions although they constituted upward of 95 percent of the staff. However, the question of the almost complete exclusion of black physicians and surgeons from the staffs of city hospitals was not a subject of investigation. On the other hand, the city administration had shown extraordinary interest in the problems of the black in housing, crime, recreation, education, and health. Playgrounds have been created, new federal housing in Harlem and other congested neighborhoods have been sponsored, new schools have been built. Health Centers have been established and public health problems vigorously attacked. However, black physicians and surgeons needed to serve the staffs of the city hospitals was a matter of chance. There was a failure to recognize the injustice of racial barriers and the consequence effect on black health. Accordingly, this failure is a tragic one for it serves

to deprive the Negro physician of that clinical
experience by which he can maintain competence and keep
pace with modern medical practice.

377.   Ray, E. S.   "Infectious Mononucleosis in the Negro."
Southern Medical Journal 37 (10) (October 1944):   543-546

A discussion of the frequency of mononucleosis in the
white race as compared to blacks.   Reports on three
cases of blacks who had the condition.   The three cases
comprise 12 percent of the cases of this disease
observed at the Medical College of Virginia Hospital
over a five year period.   The three cases were
complicated by the presence of sickle cell anemia.
Reviews the literature on infectious mononucleosis.

378.   Ray, T., Stauss, H. K. and Burch, G.
"'Angiomesohyperplasia': A Generalized Noninflammatory
Occlusive Arterial Disease," American Heart Journal 35 (1)
(January 1948): 117-125.

Describes an adult black with occlusive vascular
disease.   The disease was generalized, but affected
principally the arteries of the lower extremities and
heart.   Thermocouple and plethysmographic studies
confirmed the occlusive nature of the disease which was
further substantiated by biopsy studies.   The
etiological nature of the disease is not apparent.   A
descriptive name, "angiomesohyperplasia," has been
submitted for the syndrome.

379.   Redfern, T. C.   "The Incidence of Exophthalmic Goiter
in Negroes," Journal of the American Medical Association 75
(1) (July 3, 1920):51.

A letter to the editor that explains a case of
exophthalmic goiter in a black female and reports the
incidence of the disorder in the colored race.   Studies
admission records to determine that the incidence was
0.13 percent of white admissions and 0.03 percent of
black admissions.   Observes that "it must be remembered,
however, that whiter persons are better informed as to
the symptoms of exophthalmic goiter, and of various
symptoms of hyperthyroidism....Negroes are less likely
to describe the symptoms of such diseases, and are often
less minutely examined than white patients."

380.   Riddle, Estelle Massey.   "The Nurse Shortage--A Concern
of the Negro Public," Opportunity 25 (January 1947):22-23.

The nurse shortage was brought to a head during World
War II.   Fifty thousand civilian nurses were plunged
into the armed forces.   This caused concern to blacks
because they have never had sufficient nursing care
available to them.   Less than three percent of the
graduate registered nurses in the country are black.
Among the 1,300 accredited nursing schools in 1946, only
twenty-eight were for blacks.   Concludes that black
people must be on the alert to see that any hospital

building program will include and meet the needs of
black people. Community support is needed to assist
with a more adequate distribution of black nurses.

381. Ripley, Herbert S. "Mental Illness Among Negro Troops
Overseas." American Journal of Psychiatry 37 (January 1947):
499-511

Presents data on the incidence of mental illnesses in
black troops stationed on an isolated island in the
Southwest Pacific and comparisons made with similarly
situated white troops. Concludes that the incidence of
psychoses was found to be higher among black than white
troops and that blacks were less well equipped by virtue
of emotional and intellectual resources to adjust to war
conditions of bodily hazards.

382. Roberts, Frank L. and Crabtree, James A. "The Vital
Capacity of the Negro Child," Journal of the American Medical
Association 88 (25) (June 18, 1927):1950-1952.

A study comparing the vital capacity of a group of
normal black (1,254) and white children (1,564) living
in the same territory. Vital capacities were evaluated
on the basis of standing height, stem length, and age.
The children were grouped according to sex. The
findings suggest that black children have lower vital
capacities than white children of the same age, than
white children of the same body weight, and the same
standing height. The two groups were practically the
same when compared in terms of stem length.

383. Robinson, S., Dill, D. B., Harmon, P. M., Hall, F. G.
and Wilson, J. W. "Adaptations to Exercise of Negro and
White Sharecroppers in Comparison with Northern Whites,"
Human Biology 13 (1941): 140-158.

A study conducted jointly by the Department of
Physiology at Indiana University, The Fatigue Laboratory
at Harvard University, and the Zoology Department at
Duke University. An application of a previously
developed procedure for measuring physiological
adaptations to work. Young male sharecroppers from the
Mississippi Delta region were utilized in the study as
were young white men from Indiana University (52 and 39,
respectively). The laboratory study involved a
treadmill and various physiological measurements (e.g.,
heart rate, O_2 requirement, blood lactate and blood
sugar). The report gives the results of these tests and
makes comparisons with Northern white subjects referred
to in the earlier study.

384. Roemer, Milton I. "Special Health Problems of Negroes
in Rural Areas," Journal of Negro Education 18 (1949):
318-325.

The author identifies three impediments to adequate
health service in rural areas: economic, ecological, and
educational. It is argued that, for rural blacks, each

of these obstacles operate to a greater degree than they
do for whites. Thus, rural blacks are among the most
disadvantaged of all groups when it comes to medical
care. Points out that the shortages of medical
personnel and facilities are aggravated by blacks' lack
of purchasing power and by race discrimination. Details
reasons for shortages in personnel and facilities for
blacks in rural areas and reviews the organized health
services that are available to blacks. Briefly
describes the efforts of government programs and
voluntary agencies and argues that the nation cannot
afford dual health programs for whites and blacks.

385. Rogers, James Frederick. "Health Work in Schools For
Negroes," Journal of Negro Education 6 (1937): 519-522.

Activities directed toward improving health at black
schools are no different than those that should be used
in white schools and school officers must be committed
to the improvement of black health. Suggests that
school personnel check the school's water supply to make
sure that it is safe, provide tips on the prevention of
school fires, improving the lighting of the school room,
and train teachers to be aware of signs of disease or
physical impairment in their pupils. Stresses the
necessity of health instruction.

386. Roman, C. V. "The Negro's Psychology and His Health,"
Opportunity 2 (20) (August 1924): 237-239.

Observes that blacks' ability to think and to live would
be a fair explanatory implication of this topic and
argues that it is a peculiarity of black psychology that
three centuries of injustice and oppression have not
developed the hatred complex. Points out that nature
has built a no more effective physiological machine than
the American black at his physical best. It becomes
difficult then to answer the question of why black
mortuary statistics are the despair of health officers.
Argues that the excessively high death rate and
morbidity incidence are due to SITUATION and not to any
defect in blacks constitution or their psychology.

387. Roman, C. V. "The American Negro and Social Hygiene,"
Social Hygiene 10 (1927): 41-47.

Within limitations, a minimum standard of healthcare may
be purchased or maintained through social hygiene. The
incidence of disease among blacks is markedly increased
because of social hygiene. Morbidity and mortality is
deeply influenced by standards of personal hygiene. One
disease especially prevalent in the black population is
venereal disease. However, this is not merely a health
problem, but a moral problem. One of the basic purposes
ᶠ sociaᶫ hygiene is to advocate the highest standards
of private and public morality. If social hygiene is to
be increased, the religion of blacks must intercede.
Also the home and home training must be involved. The
home is the functional unit of any population. It is

the basic social unit. Blacks must be taught that good
health starts not with the body but with the soul.
Hygiene must be instilled in child rearing. Therefore,
black children must be taught the importance of hygiene
both physically and morally.

388.   Rosser, Curtice.   "Rectal Pathology in the Negro:
Incidence and Peculiarities," Journal of the American Medical
Association 84 (2) (January 10, 1925):93-97.

A paper read before the Section on Gastro-Enterology and
Proctology at the Seventy-Fifth Annual Session of the
American Medical Association, Chicago, June, 1924.
Reviews the rectal cases occurring at Baylor Hospital
over a five year period and the various diseases in
terms of rate of occurrence in blacks versus whites. In
general, argues that the rate of rectal disease was
equally prevalent in the two races. Cancer, pruritus,
fissure and spastic sphincter were found to be less
common in blacks. The inflammatory conditions of the
region were seen more often in blacks. Benign fibrous
stricture occurred eleven times more frequently in
blacks and was accompanied often by other manifestations
of the fibroplastic diathesis. Hemorrhoids occurred
twice as often in the white race, but had an excess of
fibrous tissue in the colored cases.

389.   Rosser, Curtice.   "Clinical Variations in Negro
Proctology: The Venereal Factor," Journal of the American
Medical Association 87 (25) (December 18, 1926):2084-2086.

A paper read before the Section on Gastro-Enterology and
Proctology at the Seventy-Seventh Annual Session of the
American Association, Dallas, Texas, April 1926.
Discusses observations of cases of rectal stricture,
which occur at higher rates in blacks than in whites.
Of black cases (26), syphilis was involved in 23
percent, gonorrhea in 23 percent, Tuberculosis in 7
percent, Chancroid in 4 percent, Operative in 4 percent,
Pellagra in 4 percent, and Undetermined in 35 percent.

390.   Rountree, L. G., McGill, K. H. and Edwards, T. I.
"Causes of Rejection and the Incidence of Defects," The
Journal of the American Medical Association 123 (1943):
181-185.

Data on rates of rejection, causes of rejection, and the
incidence of physical and mental defects among 18 and 19
year old military registrants are presented in this
paper in response to requests for information on the
physical status of this particular age group. The
sample group represented 42,273 white and 3,312 black
registrants from December, 1942 to January/February,
1943. The data were analyzed in tabular form and
indicate the rejection rates for whites, blacks and
cumulative; the causes of rejection for each race; the
incidence of defects among the registrants; and the
rejection rates by occupational group. The narrative

section of the paper explains, in depth, the findings of
the study.

391. "Sanitation and Home Improvement Highlights National
Negro Health Week in Rural Areas." Release, U.S. Department
of Agriculture. Cited in National Negro Health News, 16 (2)
(1948): 4.

   Agricultural Extension's year-round program of promoting
   better health and nutrition in rural areas was further
   emphasized during National Negro Health Week (April
   4-11) with a special drive in many communities for
   balanced diets, home improvements, and sanitation, as
   reported by T. M. Campbell and John W. Mitchell,
   Extension Service field agents of the United States
   Department of Agriculture. Holding nutrition clinics,
   painting and screening of homes, improving the water
   supply, making better provisions for sewage disposal,
   and building sanitary privies highlighted the
   observance.

392. Scheele, Leonard A. "The Health Status and Health
Education of Negroes: A General Introductory Statement,"
Journal of Negro Education 18 (1949):200-08.

   Discusses the strides that have been made in health care
   for blacks from 1929 to 1949. Life expectancy increased
   for blacks during the time period at a higher rate than
   for whites. Nevertheless, the death rates from such
   communicable diseases as pneumonia, malaria, and
   pellegra were still high for black children. Points out
   that having separate facilities for blacks or having
   inadequate sections of available facilities for use by
   blacks has had a detrimental effect on black health
   care. Also acutely felt in the black community is a
   lack of local public health services, the high cost of
   medical care, and the lack of black physicians in the
   country. Legislation such as the National Hospital
   Construction Program of 1946 and other acts granting
   federal funds to state and local governments are steps
   in the right direction.

393. Schuyler, Josephine. "Nutrition and Racial
Superiority," Crisis 49 (12) (December 1942):380-381,
397-398.

   Discusses the importance of careful nutrition. Argues
   that there is a direct relationship between proper
   nutrition and physical and mental health and that the
   health of blacks can be improved by changing their
   eating habits. Points out that "nearly 90 percent of
   the black population had diets classified as B or C.
   Concludes that "if Negro mothers really want to raise
   the status and increase the health and beauty of their
   group, they will immediately get down to the business of
   feeding their families scientifically."

394. Schwartz, Edward E. "Infant and Maternal Mortality Among Negroes," Journal of Negro Education 18 (Summer 1949): 240-250.

Discusses the decreases in black infant and maternal mortality during the past decade and half; specifically, 1933-1947. Examines the impact of medicine, public health work and social welfare programs on the decrease. Also discusses specific leading causes of black infant and maternity deaths such as stillborns and crib deaths.

395. Schwartz, Steven O. and Gore, Maurice. "Pernicious Anemia in Negroes," Archives of Internal Medicine 72 (1943): 782-785.

An analysis of the results of a study covering the period from 1931 to 1942, during which 93 blacks were found to have pernicious anemia. The study as a whole refutes the claims that pernicious anemia is rare in blacks. Concludes that pernicious anemia in blacks occurs at a rate of 36 per hundred thousand hospital admissions, contrasting with the rate of 170 per hundred thousand in Caucasians. The incidence of pernicious anemia is higher in black females than in black males.

396. Scott, Doris B. "A Negro Nurse in Industry," The American Journal of Nursing 52 (1952): 170-171.

In 1950, the House of Delegates of the American Nurses Association adopted a platform which advocated full participation of minority groups in association activities and the elimination of discrimination in job opportunities, salaries, and other working conditions. As a result of this action, Miss Doris Scott, R.N. was hired by Oak Ridge National Laboratory in Tennessee. Miss Scott was responsible for providing health education and services to approximately 3,000 persons. She also provided health education to the families of employees. Miss Scott treated both black and white patients.

397. Scott, Doris B. "The Negro Health Program at the Oak Ridge National Laboratory," National Negro Health News 16 (3) (July-September 1948):6-8.

The author was added to the Health Division of Oak Ridge National Laboratory to initiate a health program specifically directed to the black employees of the Lab. Describes the successful beginnings of the program. Following an orientation into the general health program and conferences with social welfare representatives and the local Department of Health, the author inaugurated the program during National Negro Health Week. During the inaugural week, the program consisted of a History of National Negro Health Week, daily bulletins on themes from that program and interviews with nearly all of the 160 black employees. The ensuing program consisted of a bulletin board stressing aspects of health and

sanitation, weekly orientation lectures for new
employees and a follow-up health treatment program based
on information from the initial interviews and physical
exams.

398. Scott, R. B., Jenkins, M. E. and Crawford, R. P.
"Growth and Development of Negro Infants: Analysis of Birth
Weights of 11,818 Newly Born Infants," Pediatrics 6 (3)
(September 1950): 425-431.

The analysis comprises 11,818 black newborn infants
delivered at Freedmen's Hospital during the period 1939
to 1947. There were 10,692 full term infants and 1,126
premature babies. The incidence of prematurity was 9.5
percent. The average birth weight for full term infants
was 3337 grams. The relatively higher birth weights for
black infants observed in this series is attributed in a
large measure to more favorable economic conditions
during the period of observation.

399. Seib, George A. "The M. Pectoralis Minor in American
Whites and American Negroes," American Journal of Physical
Anthropology 23 (April - June 1938): 389-417.

A study of the extent of origin and mode of insertion of
the m. pectoralis minor was undertaken in a series of
500 adults. The origin of the m. pectoralis minor
extended from the second to the fifth rib in the
majority of the cases. Additionally, the research found
that the m. pectoralis minor was more caudally in
blacks.

400. Shenehon, Eleanor. "Arkansas: Negroes Organize Social
Hygiene Education Committees and Hold Institute," Journal of
Social Hygiene 31 (5) (May 1945): 314-315.

Field Worker, Charles O. Rogers, of the American Social
Hygiene Association, organized in various parts of the
state during a series of visits, thirteen local social
hygiene committees. Communities where committees were
established included: Blytheville, Crossett, Camden,
Forrest City, Hot Springs, Little Rock, McGehee,
Marianna, Marion, Monticello, Prescott, and Texarkana.
Each committee was composed of black leaders who planned
to carry on programs. Health units and the State Health
Department supported these committees by giving advice
and guidance to their programs and by furnishing
literature, films, consultations and speakers when
possible. Summarizes program activities, membership and
participants, with references to the general welfare and
educational points of view used as criteria for adopting
a resolution recommending the establishment of a State
Social Hygiene Association.

401. Shyrock, Richard H. "Medical Sources and the Social
Historian," American Historical Review 4 (April 1936):465-8.

Discusses a study in 1841 of Josiah Nott on black
mortality rates. Nott compared the black mortality

rates of the chief eastern seaports during the first
half of the nineteenth century. He contrasted the
relatively high rates for free black in northern cities
with the relatively low rates for slaves in the southern
towns. Nott then compared the two groups (free blacks
and slaves) within the one border city of Baltimore. He
found that here, within the same climate area, free
blacks still perished more frequently than did blacks in
bondage. The physician, therefore, implied that
emancipation would be followed by increasing black
mortality.

402. "Sickle Cell Anemia: A Race Specific Disease," Journal
of the American Medical Association 133 (1) (January 4,
1947):33-34.

Observes that sickle cell anemia is a significant
disease, not because of the deformation of the cell, but
because it is a disease that is completely unique to one
race. The disease was discovered in Chicago by a black
medical student. The disease had afflicted hundreds in
the United States before it was found to originally
occur in Africa. It was later that the disease was
found to occur in other groups including Cubans,
Mexicans, Italians, Greeks, Arabs, Portuguese,
Egyptians, South Americans, and even white Americans.
The reasoning for the discovery is that these other
groups are of Mediterranean races and therefore of some
proximity to Africa. Concludes by noting that perhaps
there are other diseases that are absolutely dependent
on the presence of a specific racial characteristic.

403. Smillie, W. G. "Syphilis in the United States,
Primarily a Negro Problem," Journal of the American Medical
Association 16 (August 1943): 365-367.

Examines the serologic blood tests for syphilis from the
first two medical reports for army service between 1940
and 1942, discusses syphilis in both black and white men
in the armed services (25.2 to 1.7 percent,
respectfully) and syphilis of blacks in rural and urban
areas of the United States (4.4 and 14.6 percent,
respectfully). Florida had the largest percentage of
syphilis with 40.6 percent and Rhode Island had lowest
at 9.2 percent.

404. Smillie, W. G. and Augustine, D. L. "Vital Capacity of
Negro Race," Journal of the American Medical Association 87
(25) (December 18, 1926):2055-2058.

This study was an outgrowth of a study of hookworms in a
group of about 2,000 white and black children of school
age in South Alabama. One of the measurements obtained
was vital capacity. One of the findings was that normal
black children had markedly lower vital capacity than
white children of the same age, sex and economic status.
The results of this study as well as two other studies
suggest a racial factor. To test this assumption, the
authors studied healthy black and white males prisoners

who worked and lived together. Concludes that the vital
capacity of the black race, in both sexes, and for all
age groups studied is markedly lower than the vital
capacity for the white race. The growth curves of
weight and standing height of white and black children
correspond closely, but blacks have shorter trunk length
than whites. When vital capacity is calculated from
stem length there is less discrepancy between the vital
capacity of the two races.

405.   Smith, Alan.   "The Availability of Facilities for
Negroes Suffering from Mental and Nervous Diseases," Journal
of Negro Education 6 (1937): 450-454.

The author begins by noting the shortage of mental
hospitals for blacks in the Southern states and provides
a brief description of different kinds of mental
treatment facilities, including insane asylums and
psycopathic hospitals. Discusses improvements needed to
provide adequate mental care facilities for blacks and
the economic and social aspects of the black mental
health problem, noting that economic security would
dramatically increase black mental patients' chances of
recovery. Summarizes the facilities available to treat
blacks with mental diseases and points out that almost
all black mental patients are in public mental
institutions. Observes that in the Northern and Western
states there are no separate provisions for blacks with
mental problems, while in the border states, blacks are
cared for in separate units.

406.   Smith, Alonzo de G., Hobday, Sadie S., and Reid, E.
Lucille.   "Health Service in a Negro District." Journal of
the American Medical Association 22 (2) (1930): 68-74.

The present program at Columbus Hill, a predominantly
black New York City district, grew out of a maternity
service program; it includes supervisory maternity
service, pre-school supervision, nutrition work,
prevention of venereal disease, dental clinic, and home
visiting service. In addition, 700 applicants aged
10-35 are examined. Staff includes the following: a
pediatrician, a maternity supervisor, a nursing
supervisor, four field nurses, a dentist, a dental
hygienist, a nutritionist, a clinical worker, and a
clerk. The program operates in an eight-block area
which comprises one of the most congested areas of the
city with problems arising from poverty, ignorance,
disease, and social maladjustment. Work began in 1917
when the City Commissioner of Health invited the
Association for Improving the Conditions of the Poor to
implement an intensive educational health service
emphasizing mothers and young children. Initially, the
site was Vandebilt Clinic where the Department of Health
operated a baby health station. Presents several tables
in a discussion of nutrition services, prenatal services
and maternity services offered by the program.

407.   Smith, S. L.   "Development of a Health Education
Program for Negro Teachers," Journal of Negro Education 6
(1937): 538-547.

This article describes the progress of the development
of a health education program for black teachers in the
state of Tennessee. Discusses the final phase of a
three-step program designed to specify the differential
in mortality rates between whites and blacks in that
state, explains the reasons for the differential, and
develops a program for improving the health of blacks.
Includes a brief description of the first two studies
preceding the final phase of the project. The program
involves two complementary objectives: training
prospective teachers in health education through college
courses and training and supervising rural teachers
already in service. There are details about designing,
implementing, and evaluating the program. Early results
of the program were encouraging and it may well be
adapted in other states.

408.   Spaulding, C. C.   "Improvements in Negro Health as
Shown by Insurance Records," Opportunity 1 (12) (December
1923): 364-365.

Life insurance is based upon exact predictions
concerning the probability of human life. According to
V. D. Johnston in the article, "A New Estimate of Negro
Health" which appeared in Opportunity (September 1923),
it was noted years ago that blacks should not be insured
on the same basis as whites because of a naturally
weaker constitution. However, statistically, records
from North Carolina Mutual Life Insurance show certain
improvements in black health regarding a marked decline
in the death rate of policyholders. The improvement in
the mortality of policyholders from such diseases as
tuberculosis and typhoid fever would seem to indicate
better living and working conditions as well as
increased application of the principles of sanitation
among blacks in the states in which North Carolina
Mutual writes insurance. Suggests that an explanation
of the more favorable mortality rate experienced by
North Carolina Mutual may be found in the employment by
this company of intelligent black agents who possess in
addition to the technical knowledge necessary for the
proper selection of risks, and understanding of class
distinctions among blacks, to which white men, through
racial prejudices, have blinded themselves.

409.   Speert, Harold.   "Corpus Cancer: Clinical,
Pathological, and Etiological Aspects," Cancer 1 (November
1948):584-600.

A study of some of the circumstances associated with the
development of carcinoma of the uterine found in 255
patients. Corpus cancer is relatively rare among black
women. Colored women comprised only 4.3 percent of the
cases of carcinoma of the corpus, whereas they make up
17.9 percent of those of cervical carcinoma. Among

blacks, there have been ten times as many cases of
cervical cancer as corpus cancer.

410. St. Clair, Harvey R., "Psychiatric Interview
Experiences with Negroes," American Journal of Psychiatry
(January-June 1951-52): 113-118.

Discusses prior observations about black psychiatric
patients. Issues such as patient's aggreeableness, the
importance of dealing with hostility, and the use of
promoting self-esteem are of special significance and
different from the psychiatric study of whites.
Concludes that psychotherapy is more different with
black patients than with whites in respect to general
principles and techniques. Stresses the importance of
recognizing social status of individual patients such as
cultural levels.

411. St. Guild, C. "Tuberculosis Among Negroes: Some of the
Problems that Complicates It's Control," Journal of the
American Medical Association 101 (27) (December 30,
1933):2110-2113.

Addresses the relationship between race and
tuberculosis. Argues that economics and race combine to
make blacks unequally susceptible to tuberculosis.
Concludes that more research is necessary because of the
limited knowledge of the "epidemiologic, pathologic, and
clinical peculiarities of tuberculosis."

412. "St. Louis County Medical Society Admits Negro
Doctors." Medical Economics, March, 1950. Cited in National
Negro Health News 18 (2) (1950): 22.

The St. Louis County Medical Society voted to admit
black physicians to membership. The word "white" was
deleted from its constitution. At the same meeting, the
society admitted two black physicians to its ranks.

413. Sterling, E. B. "Physical Status of the Urban Negro
Child," Public Health Reports 43 (October 1928):2713-2774.

A study of long-range health problems created by
overcrowding and malnutrition in black children living
in inner-city areas in the American South. Based on an
analysis of the health and physical development of 5,170
black school children in Atlanta, Georgia.

414. Stern, Anne. "Wiltwyck-A Home Away From Home," Crisis
55 (11) (November 1948):330-332, 347.

A discussion of the Wiltwyck Home for Boys which is the
only state institution for black juveniles who have been
neglected by parents or have committed crimes. "The
Wiltwyck Home accepts New York City's most deprived and
neglected children, both Negro and white; children who
have been rejected by other institutions as 'hopeless'
and 'a menace to the community'" The home provides a
mental hygiene service. Every boy is interviewed by a

staff psychiatrist and given a battery of psychological
tests and a complete physical examination. Both doctors
and psychiatrists make regular visits to the home and
are on special emergency call. "An up-to-date infirmary
under the maintenance of a registered nurse is open at
all times." Medical treatment for the boys is
considered as important as the treatment of their
emotional difficulties.

415. Stevens, Rutherford B. "Racial Aspects of Emotional
Problems of Negro Soldiers," American Journal of Psychiatry
103 (1946-47):493-498.

    Discusses how to deal with emotional as well as other
    health problems of blacks for a better understanding of
    black soldiers. Argues that poor economic status, poor
    medical care and lack of education of many blacks prior
    to induction resulted in poor health with an
    accompanying increase in chronic ailments, lack of
    ambition or goal, all of which added to the difficulties
    blacks experienced in adjusting to the military.

416. Stone, Charles T. and Vanzant, Frances R. "Heart
Disease as Seen in a Southern Clinic: A Clinical and
Pathologic Survey," Journal of the American Medical
Association 89 (18) (October 29, 1927):1473-1480.

    A paper read before the Section of Practice of Medicine
    at the Seventy-Eighth Annual Session of the American
    Medical Association, Washington, D.C., May 20, 1927.
    Presents a clinical and pathologic survey of the cardiac
    cases seen at the John Sealy Hospital during the past
    seven years. Discusses detailed data concerning the
    various diseases of the heart and comparisons based on
    sex, age and race. Observes that heart disease, as a
    whole, is somewhat different in the South than in other
    parts of the country. One of the reasons is the
    proportionately larger black population in the South.
    Some findings are: 1) the incidence of heart disease is
    1.8 times as great in blacks as in the white race; 2)
    syphilitic heart disease is more frequent in the South
    than in other parts of the country due to the large
    number of blacks; 3) the rarity of angina pectoris in
    blacks was pointed out; and 4) Arteriosclerotic heart
    disease is much more common in the white race than in
    the black race.

417. Stragnell, Robert and Smith, Katherine E. "Congenital
Hemolytic Jaundice in a Negro Family," American Journal of
Medicine 1 (1) (July 1946): 53-55.

    Case report on the congenital hemolytic jaundice disease
    occurring in three siblings of a black family. The
    disease appears to be very uncommon in blacks. However,
    the case of a twenty-one year old black with typical
    hemotological findings of congenital hemolytic jaundice
    is reported. It was thought the illness represented a
    non-bacterial respiratory infection of undetermined
    etiology. A study of the family disclosed latent

hemolytic disease in his two sisters as well. Supports
the view that congenital hemolytic jaundice is rare in
blacks by examining their clinic records. Only one
black was reported with the disease during the period of
1926-1946 records, a mulatto woman with a six-year
history of jaundice.

418. "Study of Negro Health Status Reveals Progress, But
Much More Improvement Needed." Journal of Negro Education
(Summer 1949):261-271.

Between 1937-46 the black mortality rate decreased 27
percent as compared to 16 percent for whites. The
greatest cause of mortality among blacks and whites is
from heart disease, with the second being tuberculosis.
However, studies have shown that when blacks are
provided adequate medical attention, they profit better
than their white brethren. The biggest problem is that
adequate attention is not available. Hospital beds are
unevenly proportioned. Blacks have 15-20 less beds
available in proportion to their population. Black
physicians are 1 to every 3,400 blacks while white
physicians are 1 to 750 whites. Measures must be taken
to rescind these balances. More and better facilities
must be made available to blacks. But more importantly,
the black health problem must be acted on as a social
problem. Blacks are poorly fed, poorly housed, poorly
paid, poorly clothed and poorly educated. In order for
black health status to increase, black social status
must increase.

419. "Study of Negro Health Status Reveals Progress, But
Much More Improvement Needed." National Negro Health News 18
(1) (January-March 1950):18-19.

Summarizes the report on the health status of blacks in
the Summer 1949 issue of the Journal of Negro Education.
The conclusions are that progress has been made since a
similar 1937 report. However, in areas such as the even
distribution of hospital services, separate facilities
or an inadequate portion of available facilities for
blacks, shortages of black physicians and other health
personnel, there is still much room for improvement.
Points out that remedial measures were numerous in the
report and recommended the following: more and better
medical services within the reach of the population,
elimination of job discrimination, better housing, more
education, better nutrition, and elimination of
segregation and inevitably inferior facilities. Urges
that black health problems be considered American health
problems and that improvement of the general living and
social conditions of blacks will do much to improve
their health.

420. Sullivan, Maurice. "The Part of the Negro Doctor in
the Control of Syphilis," Journal of Social Hygiene 19 (8)
(November 1933): 435-444.

Discusses the great variations in data on syphilis in whites and blacks. The lowest figures are those of the United States Public Health Service's one day estimation of the disease under treatment (4.05 percent per 1000), based on the reports of 31,847 medical sources serving a mixed population of 24,498,000. New Orleans Charity Hospital Negro Male Surgical Clinic and the New Orleans Child Welfare Association Negro Maternity patients had the highest incidence of reported syphilis. Cites Turner's series in discussing the differences in the type of complications and anatomical involvement syphilis causes. Turner claims that neurorecurrences in early syphilis were twice as frequent in whites as in blacks, whereas cardiovascular syphilis, paresis and disabling forms of the central nervous system, skeletal muscle involvement, iritis, and gummata of the lymph nodes occurred predominately in blacks. In the black female, there was an extremely high rate of rectal stricture, condylomas, and eye manifestation. Contends that the well trained black physician should have the task of eliminating this disease from his own race. Black physicians and nurses are invaluable in communicating to their race the mode of transmission and precautionary measures to be dealt with in treating this disease, for they will be endowed with the ideals of scientific medical and social service, and this influence will have good effects, for his fellowmen will understand and appreciate his interest.

421. "Surgeons' Color Line." Time 52 (July 26, 1948): 61.

The American College of Surgeons, to which nearly all U.S. surgeons would like to belong has 13,000 members. One of these members is a black, Dr. Louis Tompkins Wright, a specialist in skull surgery who was admitted in 1934.

422. Swados, Felice. "Negro Health on the Antebellum Plantation," Bulletin of the History of Medicine 10 (1941):460-472.

Discusses the lack of attention given to black health care during the slavery era, including cholera, typhoid, diptheria, malaria, tetanus, sterility and the conditions that brought on all of these maladies.

423. Switzer, Paul K. "The Incidence of the Sickle Cell Trait in Negroes from the Sea Island Area of South Carolina." Southern Medical Journal 43 (1) (January 1950): 48-49.

Discusses reported incidences of sickle cell traits in various localities in the Untied States and the Sea Island area. An unusually high incidence is found in the ages from 6-10 years, 20.7 percent in males and 18.2 percent in females.

424. "Sydenham Hospital is Meeting Its Crisis," National Negro Health News 2 (June - April 1948): 5.

Dr. I. Oscar Weissmas was appointed director of Sydenham Hospital. This medical facility was built to treat crippled black children. However, the hospital services were not limited to the children. The facility served a large residential black neighborhood.

425. Sydnor, Charles S. "Life Span of Mississippi Slaves," American Historical Review 35 (1930):566-74.

Compares the life expectancy of slaves and whites in Mississippi in the ante-bellum period. Uses census data from 1850 and 1860 and an actuarial formula to determine life expectancy. Because he is concerned with the life expectancy of slaves after they were burdened with a full work load, he begins his data collection with the twenty to thirty year old age group. He discovers that at age twenty, a white person had a life expectancy of 23.72 years in 1850. The life expectancy of slaves at twenty years of age in 1850 was 22.30 years. Concludes that this was proof that slaves were not "worked to death in about seven years" in Mississippi as was claimed in some of the literature of the day. In fact, there was a strong similarity in life expectancies between slaves and whites. The author does admit that the differences in infant mortality between blacks and whites in the 1850s were highly divergent. Also notes that the disparity between black and white life expectancy grew in the 1920s (49.03 years to 40.19 years) and was proof that blacks were not treated as harshly in the ante-bellum period as many had claimed.

426. Tandy, Elizabeth C. "Infant and Maternal Mortality Among Negroes," Journal of Negro Education 6 (1937):322-49.

The author, a senior statistician for the Children's Bureau of the U.S. Department of Labor, provides a wealth of data concerning infant and maternal mortality rates among blacks from 1915 to 1935. Finds that only 20 percent of black births in the rural South (where approximately 64 percent of black births occur) were attended by physicians in 1935 (as opposed to 93.6 percent of white births nationwide). Southern states exhibit high infant mortality rates in general, but the black infant mortality rate was 80.2/1,000 live births in the rural South and 109.3/1,000 live births in the urban South (as compared to 56.0 and 68.0 for white southerners). In every category of diseases, black infants have a higher mortality rate than white infants. Black maternal mortality exceeds white maternal mortality in every section of the nation. However, the differential between black and white maternal mortality rates is less in the southern than in the northern or western states. Black infant mortality declined from about 1918 to 1935, with the largest decrease occurring in the late 1910s and early 1920s. Attributes most of the decrease in mortality rates for blacks to adaptation to the environment and general increases in healthfulness.

427.   "The American Red Cross and Negro Health."   National Negro Health News 15 (1) (January-March 1947):1-4.

Reports the increase in voluntary involvement of blacks (primarily women) in health-care programs of the American Red Cross. The stimulus for the survey of black involvement in The Red Cross programs came from the recent example of the Volunteer Nurse's Aid Corp at Mercy Hospital in St. Petersburg, Florida. In order to show their willingness to get involved and in order to improve health care for the patients at Mercy Hospital (primarily a hospital for blacks) women of the community underwent training programs and voluntarily assisted in health care at the hospital. The report includes lists of organizations and activities in both civilian and veteran health institutions in five other states as well. Areas in which the increasing activity of blacks in health aid is being felt include hospitals, clinics, schools, first aid and safety training programs, nutrition schools, and home nursing courses. All these programs were conducted under the auspices of The Red Cross.

428.   "The Health of Black Folk," Crisis 40 (2) (February 1933):31.

Discusses the causes of the high race mortality. In 1927 there were 17.3 annual deaths of blacks per thousand. In comparison to the average mortality of the nation, the black death rate was nearly two-thirds higher than that of whites. "Five diseases (tuberculosis, cancer, health disease, cerebral hemorrhage, pneumonia) together with fatal accidents, account for two-thirds of the mortality of blacks. Additionally, such ailments as typhoid fever, whooping cough, bronchitis and puerperal difficulties are also causes of black deaths. Of the above diseases, the most serious disease among blacks is tuberculosis, with pneumonia second. "Every year, 35,000 Negroes die from tuberculosis in this country and at all times, 440,000 Negroes are ill with the disease." Other causes of black deaths are venereal diseases, syphilis, cancer, organic heart disease, and death from pregnancy. The death of black children is also considerably higher than that for white children. "In 1925 the Negro infant mortality rate was 110.8 per thousand, while it was 68.3 for whites."

429.   "The National Health Council Adopts a Program for Negro Health," Journal of Social Hygiene 20 (9) (December 1934): 455-457.

The National Health Council organized a committee to direct essential studies and program activities with the purpose of meeting better the serious problem of health among American blacks. The committee's (Committee on Negro Health of the National Health Council) members were Dr. H. E. Kleinschmidt, Fr. C. Guild, Dr. Walter Clarke, Lewis Carris and Franklin O. Nichols. It was

composed of important white and black educators in the
field of student health. The committee considered its
immediate contribution to be made in directing its
efforts toward the division of black health among the
seventy colleges and teacher training schools and black
normal schools since these institutions would provide
teachers for rural areas of the South. The program
adopted for promotion by the committee is as follows:
(1) Continued essential studies in student health
services, health education, and sanitation in black
colleges; (2) Provision of consultation services for
such institutions requesting these services; (3)
Activities aimed at securing for black college students
adequate physical examinations with adequate correctives
and the institution of a system of records and
histories, instructional hygiene, and development of
interest and organizations in recreational activities;
and (4) Teacher Training Institutes to provide for
health services for student teachers, instructional work
in health education for children of elementary schools,
application of instructional work as a part of teacher
training, and guidance for setting up essential
machinery.

430.   "The Tuberculosis Problem in 1949," National Negro
Health News 18 (January - March 1950): 11-12.

Tuberculosis is a communicable disease that can be
prevented, but is was still killing nearly 1,040
Americans a week, 125 persons a day - at a rate of 1
person every 11 minutes. Tuberculosis leads all other
diseases as a cause of death among young adults from
ages 15 to 34. "Of every 12 deaths among Negroes, 11
were due to tuberculosis," Tuberculosis could strike at
any age, but the median age at which death occurred was
46. "Approximately 1,000,000 working years were lost by
those who died of tuberculosis annually." An estimated
"15,000,000 potential years of life was lost annually to
the disease." For those who survived tuberculosis, the
best treatment available was complete bed rest combined
with streptomycin.

431.   "The Year-Round and Health Week Program in St. Landry
Parish, LA," National Negro Health News 17 (July - September
1949): 6-8.

The health unit of St. Landry Parish has been
instrumental in improving the health of blacks in the
parish. The health unit participated heavily in the
National Negro Health Week geared towards educating
blacks. The St. Landry Parish Health Unit has elected
to extend the health week year round, but on a smaller
scale. Although blacks have the same health problems as
whites, their problems tended to be worse.

432.   Thompson, Raymond K., Wagner, John A. and MacLeod,
Christine M. "Sickle Cell Disease: Report of a Case with
Cerebral Manifestations in the Absence of Anemia," Annals of
Internal Medicine 29 (July-December 1948): 921-927.

The case presented is of a 20 year old colored male.
The case is of interest because there was no case
reported concerning cerebral manifestations of sickle
cell disease without anemia in which the clinical and
pathological manifestations were predominately cerebral.
"The value of routine sickling tests on all patients
presenting evidence of subarachnoid bleeding or
neurologic symptoms which might be explained on the
basis of a diffuse vascular thrombatic process has been
emphasized."

433. Tibbitts, Clark. "The Socio-Economic Background of
Negro Health Status," Journal of Negro Education 6
(1937):413-28.

Presents data on black mortality rates. Since blacks
had higher mortality rates than whites and a higher
percentage of blacks worked as unskilled laborers than
did whites, argues that socioeconomic status had a
strong correlation with high mortality rates in the
black community. Data are presented which indicate that
blacks live in less safe housing than whites; blacks
have a smaller percentage of children in high school and
college; blacks are not proportionally represented in
the health care professions; and black infant, maternal,
and general mortality rates exceed those for whites for
every disease, etc. (except for cancer, heart disease,
and diabetes, the first two of which account for a great
number of deaths). In only one study documented in this
brief literature review were blacks and whites compared
with age and income controlled. The study in which age
and income were controlled indicated that blacks in
Dayton, Ohio suffered more from serious disabilities
than whites in that city in 1934. Concludes that the
effects of increased health care availability to blacks
have, and will continue to have, a positive impact on
black health.

434. Tildon, T. T. "Cardiovascular Disease Complicating
Neurosyphilis Among Negro Veterans," Medical Bulletin of the
Veterans' Administration 13 (October 1936): 144-151.

Syphilis alone was difficult to treat. However, it was
made even more difficult when a patient developed
cardiovascular disease. Points out that cardiovascular
syphilis occurred in 70 to 90 percent of syphilitic
patients (discovered after an autopsy was performed).
Other cardio-related problems found in blacks were
hypertension and enlarged hearts. As for the question
of special susceptibility of black syphilitics to
cardiovascular disease, the author notes that further
study would be needed. However, argues that late and
inadequate treatment of syphilis were probable causes of
the higher incidence of cardiovascular disease of
syphilitic Negroes.

435. Tobey, James A. "The Death Rate Among American
Negroes," Current History 25 (November 1926):217-20.

The black population has more than doubled since 1870. The increase has been much slower for whites. However, the health of the American Negro is about thirty years behind that of the white population. The average life span of blacks is forty-six years. This is partially due to a high infant mortality rate. The high black mortality rate in cities is due to many causes, chief among which is the fact that here is a typically rural dweller placed in an unnatural environment, to which he adjusts with difficulty. Anthropological data show that the black is not inferior physically to the white, but differs in various bodily measurements, including a somewhat smaller chest size. Tuberculosis and the venereal diseases are the principal causes of death and disability among American blacks.

436. Trotter, Mildred and Lanier, Patricia T. "Hiatus Canalis Sacralis in American Whites and Negroes," Human Biology 4 (December 1945): 368-381.

Examines the extent of the Hiatus Canalis Sacralis in blacks and whites. A population of 1,225 black and white bones were studied. The report revealed that ankylosis of the first coccygeal vertebra or the entire coccyx to the sacrum (a condition which may affect the length of the hiatus) occurred significantly more in whites than in blacks, occurred at an earlier age in blacks, and its incidence increased with age significantly in white females and black males. The study also revealed that the hiatus was longer in whites than in blacks and longer in men than in females. Finally, the anteroposterior diameter of the hiatus at its apex was significantly greater in blacks than in whites.

437. "Tuberculosis Control in Pennsylvania," National Negro Health News 3 (July - September 1946): 24.

The Pennsylvania Tuberculosis Society recorded several achievements in 1945 and 1946. The society awarded scholarships to blacks engaged in or planning to do work in teaching, nursing, social work, or other community service. The scholarships enabled the recipients to take a six week summer course at the University of Michigan's School of Public Health. Additionally, contests were held in the public schools on tuberculosis and its preventive measures. The ultimate objective of Society was to stimulate active interest in blacks.

438. Turner, Edward L., "Undergraduate and Graduate Medical Education for Negroes," Journal of America1 Medical Association 116 (April-June 1941): 211-214.

Examines the number of blacks enrolled in medical schools to 1941. As of 1938-1939, only 350 medical students were black. Also examines medical association of blacks and their credibility with the medical profession. Concludes that black medical associations are becoming more credible. Outlines programs developed

by hospital facilities which have available special
courses offered to black physicians.

439. Turner, John A.   "Dental Health in Negro Colleges,"
Health Institution Yearbook (1943):237-238.

Reports findings of a dental health survey of 500 black
students at Howard University in Washington, D.C. The
survey was conducted using a questionnaire, dental
records, and X-ray films. There were a number of dental
defects found present in the student population. Of the
29 black colleges, 82.8 percent did not require
correction of the dental defects before admission and
only 10.3 percent required routine X-rays.
Recommendations for improving dental health care for
blacks include installing well-equipped dental units in
the student health departments, employing qualified
dentists who can instruct dental hygiene, mandatory
correction of dental disorders and a development of
routine methods for dental care in the future.

440. Tyson, William George.   "Negro Insurance Companies and
Syphilis Control," Journal of Social Hygiene (June 1941):
78-81.

Reports the findings of a questionnaire sent to the
medical directors of approximately 30 black insurance
companies regarding the control of syphilis. Questions
were as follows: (1) Do you make routine blood tests on
all ordinary applicants? If not, why? (2) Do you
recommend a routine blood test on all ordinary
applicants? (3) What was your average mortality rate
(ordinary and industry) in 1938 in which syphilis was a
known factor? (4) What measures have you taken in
attempt to lower this rate? (5) How can the insurance
company, in your opinion, help in lowering the high
death rate to syphilis and its sequelae? Summary: (1)
Routine blood tests are not made on all applicants, but
only when the examiner suspects a syphilitic background
or when the insured applied for amounts to $5,000. (2)
The general public is not ready to accept routine blood
tests at the discretion of the insurance examiners. (3)
Syphilis is rarely reported as such, therefore,
mortality statistics are inadequately kept by most
insurance companies. (4) Cooperation with the United
States Public Health Service Venereal Disease program
and with other public health and welfare agencies. (5)
Insurance companies agree that routine blood tests are
the most effective way to reduce the mortality rate due
to syphilis. Recommends a meeting of the National
Medical Association members to select a committee to
enter into a round table discussion of the problem.

441. "U. S. Army Utilizing the Talents of Chicago Negro
Doctors," Journal of the American Medical Association 43
(November 1942):642-643.

Many of the prominent black physicians from throughout
the country have been "drafted" for use in the care of

black soldiers overseas. A separate facility for black
soldiers to be trained has been established in Bisbee,
Arizona. Many of the black doctors drafted have been
either stationed there or at one of the black station
hospitals located overseas.

442. U.S. House of Representatives, Providing for the
Establishment of a Veteran's Hospital for Negro Veterans at
the Birthplace of Booker T. Washington in Franklin County,
Virginia. 82nd Congress, Report No. 230, pp. 5-6.

The Committee on Veterans Affairs recommended the
passage of a bill to provide for the establishment of a
veteran's hospital for black veterans in Franklin
County, Virginia. This hospital would be the third of
its kind. The Veteran's Administration at Tuskegee,
Alabama, operated a facility which cared for 2,113 black
veterans and a veteran's hospital in Mound Bayou,
Mississippi, had a bed capacity of 200. These existing
hospitals are managed and staffed completely by blacks.

443. "Underregistration: A Negro Health Problem." National
Negro Health News 16 (1) (January-March 1948):9-12.

Discusses the reasons for, facts and implications of
unregistered births and deaths in the United States
particularly as they pertain to blacks. Points out that
unregistered births are particularly a problem among
blacks in the rural South. Among rural southern whites,
1 birth in 6 is unregistered whereas among rural
southern blacks, 1 in 4 is unregistered. Explanations
provided are isolation, fewer taxable resources and
below standard education in rural areas of the South.
Although conditions have improved since 1940 due to the
war years' emphasis on birth certificates required for
work, to prove dependency benefit claims for military
children and the heroic efforts of state registrars of
vital statistics. No data on the improvement are yet
available. Explains the value of birth certificates
under two categories, 1) as a legal document proving
certain facts and 2) as a statistical record providing
data for planning and executing health and welfare
programs. Birth certificates are essential for entering
school, establishing age (for work papers, social
security, old age pensions), and for proof of parentage
for insurance and inheritance purposes. Death
certificates are necessary for insurance and inheritance
purposes and for providing valuable statistical records.
These death records help states obtain grant-in-aid
funds for hospitals and clinics. They also provide
valuable information for fighting tuberculosis or other
dangerous diseases.

444. Usilton, Lida J. "A Tentative Death Curve for Acquired
Syphilis in White and Colored Males in the United State,"
Venereal Disease Information 18 (7) (July 1937): 231-232.

Explores the death rate for acquired syphilis among
white and negro males compared to the death rate among

white and black males not infected. Finds that the
death rates for white males between the ages of 30 and
75 years with acquired syphilis are shortened
considerable over those found in the noninfected white
population. Insufficient data made proof of a higher
death rate among white males above the age of 75 years
with acquired syphilis an impossibility. The life
expectance of white males between the ages of 30 and 60
years with acquired syphilis is shortened by seventeen
percent. Among black males with acquired syphilis, the
death rate was considerably higher than the same
uninfected population from 30 years of age to death.
Concludes by observing that black males between the ages
of 30 and 60 years with acquired syphilis have a life
expectancy thirty percent shorter than the general
population.

445. Valien, Preston et al. "Attitudes of the Negro Mother
Toward Birth Control," American Journal of Sociology 55
(November 1949):279-83.

Discusses black attendance practices at a birth control
clinic in Nashville in 1940. One hundred and forty-six
mothers were surveyed. The Nashville Public Health
Nursing Council offered free birth control to needy
families and sponsored several birth control clinics.
Some 98 or 67.1 percent of the mothers never attended
the clinics. Of the 48 who did, 14 or slightly more
than one-fourth had attended before their 1940
pregnancy. Several of these fourteen stated that they
had improperly used the birth control. Sixty-nine had
favorable attitudes toward birth control, while 67
expressed disfavor. Their criticism mainly revolved
around the sinfulness of birth control. A large
percentage of the mothers favoring birth control were of
urban birthplace. Mothers having twelve or more years
of schooling also reacted favorably to birth control.

446. Van Ingen, Phillip. "Why Negro Babies Die?"
Opportunity 1 (7) (July 1923): 195.

The author, Secretary of the American Child Health
Association, discusses comparative data on infant
mortality among various racial groups. The average
infant mortality during the period 1916-1920 for native
born white Americans was 40.6 percent. The black group
stood at the peak with an infant mortality average 129
percent higher than the native-born group. It is
suggested that after the first month of life, disease
and death are due to the effects of a "germ-laden"
atmosphere. The brunt of health efforts, therefore, are
expected to fall upon living conditions to which
children are exposed and upon the care provided for
them. Another important cause of infant mortality among
blacks are diseases classed as "developmental". These
are congenital malformations, premature and congenital
debility resulting from the lowered physical condition
and habits of the mother's living before childbirth.
Offers the following suggestion to the black population:

"When communities appreciate that it is cheaper and
better to spend money in preventing disease than in
curing it, and that to develop personal health and
health habits is true patriotism, we shall accomplish
our end".

447. Vinson, Porter P. "Incidence of Esophageal Disease in
Negroes." Southern Medical Journal 38 (7) (July 1945):
452-453.

A racial comparison of incidence of Esophageal Disease
at the Medical College of Virginia Hospital. Compares
blacks to the whites and the number of cases. Observes
that the lesions of the esophagus which may have their
origin in congenital abnormalities are encountered more
frequently in the white than in the black patient.
Concludes from recent studies that congenital
deformities, which occur more frequently in white than
in black people, may be the result of the presence of
the Rh factor in the black race and that the presence of
the Rh in the black may be the reason for the difference
in the occurrence of certain esophageal lesions in black
and white persons.

448. "Vital Statistics (Negroes Hard Hit by Tuberculosis),"
American Journal of Public Health 24 (1934): 154.

Nearly one-fourth of all deaths from tuberculosis in
Illinois were among blacks. Mortality from tuberculosis
among blacks were six times greater than among whites.
The mortality rate tuberculosis among blacks in Illinois
were more than twice the death rate from tuberculosis
among blacks in Arkansas, Florida, Georgia, Louisiana,
Mississippi, and South Carolina. Furthermore, the
process toward eradicating tuberculosis in Illinois had
been much less among blacks than among whites. During
the last ten years, the tuberculosis death rate in
Illinois had declined only 19 percent for blacks while
among whites death declined 45 percent.

449. Wagner, Phillip S. "A Comparative Study of Negro and
White Admissions to the Psychiatric Pavilion of Cincinnati
General Hospital," American Journal of Psychiatry 45
(1938):167-83.

The author, a psychiatrist from Towson, Maryland,
designed an experiment to determine whether there are
differences between blacks and whites in regard to
mental illness. Utilizes data from a hospital in
Cincinnati that accepts mental patients and compares
findings with a previous study done in New York City.
The data reveal that blacks are disproportionately
represented as mental patients in relation to treatment
for all mental illnesses except for those catagories
identified as "involutional" and "hysteria." However,
more black mental illness could be explained away by the
presence of syphilis in the central nervous system. The
data on New York City did not reveal any discrepancies
with the Cincinnati data vis-a-vis black/white

incidences of mental illnesses. Concludes that after examining the files of each of the Cincinnati patients there was no qualitative difference between incidences of mental illness in blacks and whites that cannot be explained by environmental rather than biological factors.

450. Walker, Helen E. The Negro in the Health Profession (Charlottesville: University of Virginia, 1949).

This work examines the role of blacks in the medical profession in the mid-1900's. Suggests that prior to this time, the black's entry into the health profession was affected by economic, cultural and educational factors. The book's thesis centers around determining the status of blacks in the medical profession in regard to (1) the obstacles created by segregated training facilities; (2) the degree of discrimination in the training of blacks; (3) utilization of black professionals in the nation's health program; and (4) place of blacks in the future of medicine. Of the total 176,000 physicians in the U.S. in 1945, approximately 4,000 or 2 percent were black. One reason for the lack of black physicians was lack of adequate training facilities. The first black's claim to a stake in the medical profession came with the opening of two training facilities, Howard Medical School in 1869 and Meharry Medical College in 1876. Until this time most blacks received their medical training abroad or as the result of extended apprenticeships. Another factor which limited the entry of black in the medical profession was discrimination. The average black physician generally lacked the opportunity to train and take part in the medical care of his patients. He was assumed to be inferior by whites. This impeded the growth of competent black physicians. Also, black physicians, were only involved in the care of other blacks. Modern medical techniques and equipment were reserved for the white segment of the population. Concludes that the future of blacks in the medical profession rested in the Hospital Survey and Construction Act, which constructed much needed hospitals and gave the black physician a chance to work with modern techniques; regional education; and the President's Committee on Civil Rights. It should be noted that the President's Committee on Civil Rights refused special entry of the black into the American Medical Association.

451. Walsh, Groesbeck and Pool, Robert M. "Disease and the Negro," The American Journal of Medical Sciences 196 (August 1938): 252-261.

Observations of the Negro's body depicted certain differences among the black and white races. These changes go beyond surface color differences. Studies found one thing for sure; that blacks experienced a higher incidence of contracting diseases, particularly respiratory ailments. Treatment for the black was a rare element, especially in the South. The author

claims educating the black in body and social hygiene
was needed to help combat diseases.

452. Walsh, Groesbeck and Pool, Robert M. "Disease and the
Negro: Thyroid Involvements," The American Journal of Medical
Sciences 199 (2) (February 1940): 255-261.

Sparse literature on thyroid disease in blacks has led
to the assumption that the disease is rare among the
colored. This study casts doubt on this assumption.
Describes incidence of the disease in Southern blacks.
From a comparison of whites living in the same area, the
authors conclude that the incidence of the disease shows
no difference between the two races. The authors are
unable to determine why blacks have a normal incidence
of this disease while diseases of similar origin are
rare among blacks. Concludes that accessibility to
inspection and the manner in which the symptoms of the
disease become portions of the host's personality as
factors which cannot be ignored.

453. Washington, Forrester B. "Health Work for Negro
Children," Opportunity 3 (33) (September 1925): 264-265.

Discusses mortality rates of black infants and other
data that supports his contention about the importance
of the country's need for a stronger and more healthful
younger generation of blacks. For example, The
Children's Hospital of Philadelphia reported
still-births of blacks in large numbers because of
contracted pelvics in black mothers, a condition due to
rickets in childhood. The lives of children of such
mothers could have been saved if the mothers had enjoyed
proper health care in their youth. Outlines health
conditions among black children throughout the country,
including New York City, Washington, D.C., Baltimore,
Birmingham and others. Notes the causes of high
mortality rates of black children: (1) the economic
status of the family as determined by the father's
earning power; (2) the lack in many sections of health
work for blacks, particularly for black children; and
(3) the ignorance of black parents, not inherent but due
to the denial of decent schooling in many sections of
the South.

454. Weber, Elmer W. "Heart Clinic for Children of
Evansville, Indiana Schools," National Negro Health News
(January - March 1946): 4-5.

Periodic health examinations were conducted for children
in the Evansville public schools by the Health
Department. The health examinations were implemented by
school medical advisors who were employed by the Board
of Education. As a result of the examinations, heart
ailments were found to be prevalent at three black
schools. The medical advisor consulted with other
medical professionals which lead to a heart clinic at
the target schools.

455.   Weber, Francis J.   "Tuberculosis and the Negro,"
National Negro Health News 16 (January - March 1948): 2.

In 1945, for the first time in history, "Negro
tuberculosis deaths fell below 100 per 1000 population."
The new figure was 98 death per 1000 population. This
was especially meaningful because 30 years earlier, the
death rate was four times as great. However,
encouraging as the trend was, the author notes that
America was guilty of complacency; the county seemed
satisfied with the present tuberculosis control measures
among blacks. Records show that blacks comprised only
10 percent of the population, but suffered 25 percent of
all tuberculosis deaths. Since tuberculosis progressed
so rapidly and deadly in blacks, the author argues that
early case finding was the key to saving black lives.
Suggests an intensification of control measures in areas
where tuberculosis hazards are greatest. Points out
that facilities for treatment and isolation of
tuberculosis are grossly inadequate to treat the needs
of blacks. Concludes that resistance building measures
should be employed to help combat tuberculosis in
blacks.

456.   Wedum, Arnold G. and Wedum, Bernice G.   "Rheumatic
Fever in Cincinnati in Relation to Rentals, Crowding, Density
of Population, and Negroes," American Journal of Public
Health 34 (October 1944):1065-1070.

Emphasizes the importance of poverty and crowding in the
genesis of rheumatic fever. However, poverty and
crowding are only signposts pointing to a more
fundamental epidemiological principle. While poverty
itself is not the factor contributing to the high
incidence of the fever in the poor, poverty causes the
factors which do influence the contraction rate: 1)
crowding and 2) inability to control the micro-climate.
It is not always possible for the poor man to rest
whenever he is tired, get warm when he is cold, and keep
dry when it is raining. These factors reduce the
person's power to resist disease such as this type of
fever.

457.   Wells, Katherine Z.   "Health Education in Harlem,"
Opportunity 1 (12) (December 1923): 361-363.

Outlines the activities of the Harlem Tuberculosis
Committee of the New York Association, organized in 1922
by Harlem citizens in conducting an active local
campaign against the disease in Harlem. The financial
support for a neighborhood educational and information
center came from the general funds of the New York
Tuberculosis Association, secured yearly in its
city-wide sale of Christmas Seals. The center served in
the capacity of a connecting link between the public
health resources of the city and community, the
volunteer and professional services of the local
physicians, the interest of local laymen and the general
population of Harlem. Whenever necessary, personal

service was given to put the individual in touch either
with a physician or with the proper clinic or public
agency. The ambition of the Committee was to help bring
the death rate down to that of the general population
within the next decade.

458. Wenger, O. C. "A Wassermann Survey of the Negroes of
the Cotton Plantation in Mississippi," Venereal Disease
Information 10 (7) (July 1929): 281-287.

   The purpose of this study is to determine the incidence
   of syphilis in fourteen cotton plantations in
   Mississippi. Incidence of syphilis infection is
   measured by Wassermann tests. The public health threat
   due to syphilis among rural blacks in the South is also
   measured. The results of the study indicated that
   approximately twenty-five percent of blacks tested
   showed positive Wassermann and that syphilis in the
   Southern States may be a more important health problem
   than malaria, pellegra, or hookworm. The high incidence
   of syphilis in the rural Southern black is of particular
   concern to plantation owners and the State Board of
   Health. These parties demonstrated a desire to develop
   some practical plan to treat the massive health problem
   created by syphilis in the Southern rural black.

459. Wenger, O. C. "The Pitt County, N.C. Demonstration for
the Control of Syphilis Among the Rural Negro Population,"
Venereal Disease Information 10 (October 20, 1930): 441-448.

   Discusses the possibility of mass control of syphilis in
   selected population areas. In particular, the
   demonstration in Pitt County, North Carolina was aimed
   at determining the number of positive Wassermanns in a
   group of "unselected" rural blacks representing all ages
   and sexes. An additional purpose was to provide
   treatment to the positive syphilitic blacks. The
   results showed a large number of cardiovascular syphilis
   cases. Additionally, enlarged thyroids were found to be
   present in black females, but second and primary
   syphilis was rare. The treatment of those blacks with
   syphilis included "energetic treatment for the early
   cases, conservative treatment for the later cases, and
   palliative treatment for the nerve cases."
   Neoarsphenamine intravenously given and mercury by the
   "belt method" were the routine treatments given to
   blacks.

460. Wenger, O. C. and Heller, J. R. "Untreated Syphilis in
the Male Negro: A Comparative Study of Treated and Untreated
Cases," Venereal Disease Information 17 (9) (September 1936):
260-265.

   This study attempts to determine differences in
   morbidity between untreated and treated cases of
   syphilis in the adult black male. Uses clinical and
   laboratory findings of 399 adult black males with
   untreated syphilis and 201 nonsyphilitic adult black
   males in comparable age groups. The results indicate

that morbidity in the black male with untreated syphilis
is much greater than morbidity in the black male with
treated syphilis and that treatment for syphilis
prevents all forms of clinical relapse for the first
fifteen years of the infection. Cardiovascular and
nervous system involvements by the disease were two to
three times as common in the untreated syphilis group as
in a comparable group receiving less than adequate
treatment.

461. "West Virginia State College Completes Second Health
Education Workshop." National Negro Health News 14 (2)
(April-June 1946):1-6.

Describes the Second Summer Health Education Workshop
held at West Virginia State College, Institute, June
17-29, 1946. The Workshop was designed "especially for
teachers who through their work in the various schools
and communities discover certain problems of health in
which they need guidance." The Workshop considered six
health-related areas of study: Nutrition, Social
Hygiene, Dental Health, Health Inspection and
Communicable Disease Control, Safety and Accident
Prevention, and Materials and Methods of Health
Education in Elementary and Secondary Schools. The
participants are listed by group and brief summaries are
made for each group. Highlights of the suggestions for
improved health care in these areas are: (1) in this
time of food shortage, meeting children's nutritional
needs is a matter of education and economics (with
Federal Government money for the school lunch programs);
(2) placing emphasis on nutrition and dental hygiene;
(3) the establishment of a school health council to
identify and address health needs in the schools; (4)
the education of youth in ways of forming habits for
personal and group security to eliminate venereal
disease along with more guidance from parents and
schools in matters of sex; and (5) the coordination of
schools and civic organizations to educate teachers and
students in accident prevention using innovative
education techniques. Concludes by describing a special
lecture on safety in mines, field trips to the State
Department of Health and the City Water Works, a list of
the social events, and a list of the Workshop's Director
and Consultants.

462. Wilber, Ray Lyman. "Negro Cooperation in the White
House Conference," Opportunity 8 (11) (November 1930):
328-330.

The author, Secretary of the Interior, discusses the
importance of the participation of black experts in
child care in the work of the White House Conference on
Child Health and Protection. The White House Conference
was the first Presidential Commission to study the
health of children in America on a national scale, from
social, economic, and humane points of view. It was the
first to acknowledge the positive cooperation and
participation of black experts in child care. The

purpose of the Conference was to establish irreducible
minimum standards for the health, education and work of
the American child. Results were shown in the
development of legislation and administrative practice
in the various states. During the sessions, reports
were given covering present procedures in medical
service, public health service and administration,
education and training, care of the handicapped child,
and recommendations for improving them. Notes that
experts were contributing largely to the conference from
their understandings and experience. It was expected
that through the universality of the scope of the
Conference more opportunities for black experts to serve
the black race would be created.

463. Williams, E. Y. "The Incidence of Mental Disease in
the Negro," Journal of Negro Education 6 (1937):377-392.

Presents data on comparative rates of mental illness
between blacks and whites. The data are drawn from a
number of different studies. The first group of data
show that mental illness has been rising in the black
population from 1860 to 1890. In New York City in
1929-31, incidences of mental illness in blacks were
twice as high (proportionally) as that of whites.
However, the author displays data that indicate that
white rates of mental illness were proportionally higher
than black mental illness rates in 1910, 1922, and 1923.
The author also compares types of mental illnesses and
their relative frequencies of occurrence in whites and
blacks. Controlling for economic status, the author
finds that 55.5 percent of blacks and 27.0 percent of
whites were admitted to state hospitals in 1933. Only
3.1 percent (for blacks) and between 5.6 percent and
12.3 percent (for whites) of those in the "comfortable"
category were admitted to state hospitals. Finally,
incidences of admission were twice as high for both
blacks and whites living in urban, as opposed to rural
areas. Concludes that high incidences of mental illness
in blacks can be attributed primarily to marginal
economic safety and to black migration to urban
environments. Suggests future research control for
opportunity differences, state versus private
hospitalization, educational differences, and etc.

464. Williams, E. Y. and Carmichael, C. P. "The Incidence
of Mental Disease in the Negro," The Journal of Negro
Education 18 (Summer 1949): 276-282.

Investigates whether there has been a high incidence of
mental disease among blacks and notes that previous
research indicates that the incidence of mental disease
among blacks has increased. However, several factors
call validity of current research into question: no
private institution in the U.S. will accept a black as a
mental patient; in the South it has been the practice to
admit only the most severely mentally ill blacks; and no
scientific studies conducted to date show relationship
of social and economic barriers due to racism on the

incidence of mental illness among blacks. Concludes
that increased urbanization of blacks, as well as
certain environmental, economic and social factors
appear to be related to increasing incidence of mental
illness among blacks.

465. Williams, Elaine, Harris, Elsie and Charles, Hilda.
"Project for National Negro Health Week," The American
Journal of Nursing 50 (April 1950): 245-246.

The nursing students at Freedmen's Hospital cooperated
with health agencies in the District of Columbia for the
improvement of health in their community. The junior
nursing students at Freedmen's set up a series of health
education exhibits as a class project. The lobby of the
hospital was used to display the exhibits. The exhibits
included booths on social hygiene, tuberculosis,
housing, nutrition, child care, and adult hygiene.
Various types of literature were available for residents
to take home.

466. Williams, Philip F. "Maternal Welfare and the Negro,"
The Journal of the American Medical Association 132 (November
1946):611-614.

Points out that while outstanding progress has been made
in the area of reducing deaths per 10,000 live births,
the outlook for black mothers is not good. Black death
rates for babies are double that of white babies.
Studies have shown that blacks do not face any intrinsic
hazard because of their race, but if they had received
adequate health care, there probably would be no
discrepancies between blacks and whites. The relatively
poor economic status of blacks seriously influences the
maternity situation in an adverse way. Because of poor
hygenic surroundings, blacks have a lower resistance to
infection and disease.

467. Winters, Jet C. "The Relation of Human Nutrition to
the Social and Economic Conditions of the South," Journal of
the American Dietetic Association 16 (1940): 215-221.

Postulates that the per capita income for the South is a
strong indication that the dietary intake of southerners
(black and white) is below that of those in other
regions. The per capita income of the richest Southern
state is still lower than any other state in any other
region. Thus, the food items that are within the means
of purchase of those in the South are typically lower in
nutritional value than the food items purchased by other
individuals in other areas. This dilemma is heightened
in the black communities of the South. There is even a
lower per capita income among blacks in the region and
thus, the blacks were unable to purchase food items of
higher nutritional value. Nutrition education is also
cited as a means to help those with minimal income.

468. Wright, Louis T. "Cancer As It Affects the Negro,"
Opportunity 6 (June 1928):169-170, 187.

Discusses and summarizes the occurrence of cancer in
peoples around the world frequently citing studies and
conclusions from numerous physicians. Several factors
once considered significant causes of cancer in blacks
can now be refuted, i.e. climate, diet, changes in
environment and others. One suggestion the author does
not dismiss is that the incidence of cancer is higher in
proportion to the degree of civilization of a people.
Applied to blacks in America, the author argues that
this seems to explain the increasing number of cases of
cancer among blacks. To substantiate this observation,
the author cites data (taken from Dublin) which indicate
the increase of cancer among blacks. Concludes that
cancer is common among American blacks, mortality among
blacks is increasing and will likely continue to
increase, it is not race related and there will be a
greater need for the education of blacks in cancer
control.

469. Wright, Louis T. "The Negro Physician," <u>The Crisis</u>
(September 1929): 305-306.

About 7,000 black physicians provide health care, mostly
to black patients. Most practice east of the
Mississippi. Since World War I more blacks and
physicians live in the North. Black doctors migrated in
order to increase scientific opportunities and to
improve economic conditions. Contrary to the prevailing
opinion in this country, the average black physician has
received the same degree of training as physicians of
other races. Howard University in Washington, D.C., and
Meharry Medical College in Nashville, Tennessee educate
most black physicians. Both are rated a Class "A" by
the American Medical Association; together they graduate
about three-fourths of black doctors. The remaining
one-fourth graduate from white medical colleges in the
East and Middle West. One-third of the black medical
graduates are either college graduates or have completed
an accredited premedical course. Interns receive
training at several black institutions which are named.
In addition, Cook County Hospital of Chicago and New
York's Harlem Hospital and Bellevue Hospital afford
black doctors the opportunity to train. About
one-fourth of the black physicians have interned prior
to practicing medicine. Opportunities for postgraduate
training are meager. Although some blacks have taken
special summer courses at Harvard and Columbia, they are
not welcomed in most postgraduate schools, especially in
clinical courses. As a result, many black physicians go
to Europe to study - a sad indictment of American
institutions, according to Dr. Wright. About the same
percentage pass and fail the State Board examinations as
other racial groups except in Florida and Mississippi
where it is almost impossible for a black graduate of a
Northern medical school to pass even though he has
easily done so in a Northern state. Hospital
connections available for licensed graduates are offered
by the so-called "colored hospitals" which have about an
equal number of colored and white physicians, but

entirely colored internes. Larger Northern hospitals
are gradually employing Negroes. Names of hospitals
which do so are given. The role of the National Medical
Association is increasing opportunities for training and
research as described. The remainder of Dr. Wright's
article deals with the role of Negro physicians.
Although most colored physicians engage in general
practice, many served as medical officers during the
war, especially with the 92nd division, which
distinguished itself. Commendations are quoted. Many
Negro physicians are quite distinguished; three serve as
administrators of large hospitals, several teach in
northern universities and many specialize in various
fields including surgery. In addition, many are
involved in research, which knows no color line.

470.   Young, Martin D. "Induced Malaria in Negroe Paretics
With Mapharsen and Tryparsamide," Public Health Reports 54
(33) (August 18, 1939):1509-1511.

Discusses the treatment of malaria in black patients.
One treatment involved the use of Mapharsen, an arsenic
compound that had been successfully used in the
treatment of syphilis. Marpharsen had been discovered
as a treatment of malaria because it stopped the chills
and fever. This drug did take away the effects of
malaria, but it did not kill the malaria parasites as
they were still present in patients some nine months
after treatment. Concludes that even though the drug
could possibly be used for the treatment of both malaria
and syphilis, but because it did not get rid of the
parasite, patients could be released from hospitals and
still be carriers of the malaria parasite.

3

THE LITERATURE OF THE
MID-TWENTIETH CENTURY,
1951–1960

471. Atchison, Calvin O. "Use of the Wechsler Intelligence
Scale for Children with Eighty Mentally Defective Negro
Children," American Journal of Mental Deficiency 60 (2)
(October 1955):378-379.

> Data were obtained on 80 feeble-minded black boys and
> girls in order to determine if there was a difference
> between Verbal and Performance IQ scores obtained on the
> Wechsler Intelligence Scale for Children (WISC). An
> analysis of the scores yielded significant results with
> the verbal mean exceeding the performance mean. These
> results indicated that equal Verbal and Performance IQ's
> on the WISC may not be characteristic for black children
> classified as familial defectives. Further work is
> needed to see if similar results would be obtained for
> larger samples of children falling in this category.

472. Banks, L. Otto and Scott, Roland B. "Thalassemia in
Negroes: A Report of a Case of Cooley's Anemia in a Negro
Child," Pediatrics 11 (6) (1953):622-627.

> Originally thought to occur only in peoples of
> Mediterranean origin, the authors report finding seven
> cases of Cooley's anemia in Negroes reported in the
> American literature. The case they present is the
> youngest to be reported. They discuss the diagnostic
> studies and the treatment procedures. Of note is the
> genetic study the authors conducted. Both parents were
> described as having typically Negroid features and no
> history of Caucasian admixture. They studied family
> members for several generations and found abnormalities
> in the blood of the patient's mother, father, maternal
> grandmother, maternal great-grandfather, maternal aunt,
> uncle, and paternal grandmother. Although the authors
> cannot ruleout unknown and remote admixture, they
> conclude that the concept of Cooley's disease as
> occurring only in Mediterranean peoples must be revised.
> Further, the results of this study suggest that Cooley's
> disease may be more common in the Negro population than
> previously realized.

473. Bartfield, Harry. "Gout in Negroes," Journal of the
American Medical Association 154 (4) (January 23, 1954):
334-336.

Discusses Gout and its relation to blacks. Concludes
that Gout is a disease rarely seen in women. It is said
to occur infrequently in blacks, but a number of cases
have occurred in clinics where blacks are in large
numbers. It was never reported as appearing in a black
woman until 1953. The article looks specifically at a
black woman who had Gout over a period of 6 years.

474. Bass, David E., Iampietro, P. F., and Buskirk, E. R.
"Comparison of Basal Plasma and Blood Volumes of Negro and
White Males." Journal of Applied Physiology 14 (5)
(September 1959): 801-803.

Basal plasma and blood volumes of seventeen American
black soldiers were compared with those of seventeen
white soldiers. Both groups were matched with respect
to height, weight, and age. Daily activity and diet
were the same for all men for two weeks prior to
measurement. All measurements were obtained in the
morning. Although both groups displayed the same
hematocrits (packed cell volumes), the authors note that
blacks had smaller amounts of both plasma and
circulating red cell volume. The author's, however,
find it difficult to attribute such differences directly
to race. Although black soldiers have had a reportedly
greater susceptibility to cold injury, the authors
cannot draw conclusions regarding the role of
differences in basal blood volume. The lack of
laboratory control over the soldiers earlier lives
necessarily limits any claim of racially based
distinctions.

475. Beddoe, Harold L. "Barium Ganuloma of the Rectum,"
Journal of the American Medical Association 154 (9) (February
27, 1954): 746-748.

Discusses Barium Granuloma of the Rectum and
specifically a case of a 53 year old black man. Focuses
on the cause and effects of barium being deposited in
the rectal wall of this black and traumatic injuries
caused by perforation. The presence of a rectal polyp,
hemorrhoids, or a fissure increases the possibility of
trauma to the rectal wall. Concludes that this is the
first case that appears to have been reported in both
the black race and human race in general.

476. Bennett, H. D. and Lyle, A. B. "Temporal Arteritis
Occurring in a Negro," American Heart Journal 42 (3)
(September 1951): 447-452.

A case of temporal arteritis is presented. This is the
first case reported in a member of the black race. The
clinical course is characteristic with persistent
low-grade fever, inflammation of the temporal arteries,
and relief of pain by severance. The black patient had
an old history of syphilis. Definite arteriosclerotic
changes are present in the patient including coronary
insufficiency and funduscopic changes. The course was
benign with complete subsidence of symptoms referable to

temporal arteritis, but persistence of symptoms of
moderate myocardial insufficiency and coronary artery
disease, suggesting involvement of multiple arteries.
No eosinophilic or polymorphonuclear leucocytes were
present. Scattered giant cells were detected.

477. Berman, L. B. "The Nephropathies of Sickle-Cell
Disease," Archives of Internal Medicine (103) (1959):
602-606.

A case report which discusses the previously over looked
renal complications of sickle-cell disease and trait,
which are called "nephropathies." The subject of the
case study is a 9 year old Black patient with hemoglobin
S. Discusses the chronological steps first reviewing
the previous medical history of the patient and the
methods of treatment used. The conclusion reached was
that corticotropin (ACTH) administration was without
significant effect.

478. Blassingille, B. "Rehabilitation of Negro
Post-Leukotomy Patients," Journal of Nervous and Mental
Disease 121 (January-June 1955): 527-533.

Discusses the post-leukotomy rehabilitation program at
the Veteran's Administration Hospital, Tuskegee,
Alabama. Evaluates the program critically, compares it
with similar programs published in the literature, and
notes those cultural, social, and economic problems
peculiar to the rehabilitation of the black leukotomized
veteran.

479. Boyles, Paul W. and Currie, Jane. "Classic Hemophilia
in a Negro Infant," The American Journal of Medical Sciences
235 (4) (April 1958): 452-454.

Addresses the absence of hemophilia in the black race.
The author points out that at the time of the study, the
disease had been reported only twenty-nine times in
blacks. The introduction of the thromboplastin
generation test in 1959 made it possible to classify
hemophiliac diseases as deficiencies of either plasma,
serum or platelet factors. This particular study looked
at one black infant who suffered from hemophilia due to
specific deficiency of the plasma factor,
anti-hemophiliac globulin. This case was verified by
the thromboplastin generation test and proves that
hemophilia can occur in the American black, possibly
with greater frequency than indicated from earlier
literature.

480. Bullock, William H., Johnson, J. B. and Davis, T.
Wilkins. "Hemophilia in Negro Subjects," Archives of
Internal Medicine 100 (1957): 759-764.

Prior to this study, it was thought that hemophilia
among blacks was quite rare. This paper, however,
presents 14 cases of hemophilia in black subjects, and
states that one possible reason for the small number of

reported causes in black subjects is that these cases
have been unsuspected or inadequately studied. The
study is of particular interest because "some of these
cases first seen in childhood have been followed for 11
years, into young adult life, with a careful study of
the changes which occurred with increasing age."
Concludes that this disorder may occur with greater
frequency in blacks than is reflected in the medical
literature.

481.   Burch, G. "The High-Pork Diet of the Negro in the
Southern United States," Archives of Internal Medicine 100
(1957): 859-860.

Begins with the observation that "dietary factors among
peoples of different races and geographic locations have
often been incriminated as a cause for variations in
racial distribution of certain diseases." Points out
that there is "a higher incidence of hypertension in the
Negro than in the white man of the Southern United
States." The research objective was to obtain a general
impression of the amount of pork included in the diet of
the average black of the Southern United States, using a
representative sample of Charity Hospital patients.
Concludes that "the factors in pork responsible for the
symptoms of hypertension remain to be identified."
However, more extensive analysis should provide "an
interesting, and perhaps enlightening study."

482.   Carr, Richard D. and Levine, Robert. "Systemic Lupus
Erythematosus of Long Duration." A.M.A. Archives of
Dermatology 81 (January-June 1960): 427-431.

Describes a 51 year old black woman admitted into
Lackland Air Force Base Hospital in October, 1957
complaining of blindness. The patient appeared older
than her age and to be chronically ill. Scattered over
her scalp, face, upper back, upper chest, neck, and arms
were discrete and irregular areas of depigmentation,
hyperpigmentation, alopecia, atrophy, follicular
plugging, erythema, and telangiectasis. The authors
comment upon the patient's apparently 23 year long
history of systemic lupus erythematosus, a notably long
survival period with such a disease. The patient was
treated with surgery, radiation, and corticosteriods,
and subsequently discharged from the hospital.
Corticosteriod treatments of decreasing amounts were
continued on an outpatient basis.

483.   Chapman, John R., "Sickle Cell Anemia," Journal of
the American Medical Association 151 (January-April 1953):
965.

Reports on a 24-year-old black female patient who has
sickle cell anemia and requires up to 15 blood
transfusions daily. Treatment is not effective.
Splenectomy is of no value because the adult spleen is
usually atrophied.

484. Chernoff, Amoz I. "On The Prevalence of Hemoglobin D
In The American Negro." Blood 10 (October 1956): 907-909.

A study of 1000 midwestern blacks which found that .4
percent carried hemoglobin D. This was unusual because
the only other few instances of this hemoglobin were
found in white individuals. With rare exceptions,
hemoglobin S (sickle-cell) and hemoglobin C are limited
to people with black ancestry. These tests are
important because these abnormal hemoglobins were the
first to cross racial lines.

485. Christopherson, W. M. and Parker, J. E. "A Study of
the Relative Frequency of Carcinoma of the Cervix in the
Negro," Cancer 13 (4) (July/August 1960):711-713.

A group of black women compared to a group of Caucasian
women as to the prevalence of squamous carcinoma of the
cervix and related cervical atypias. Both groups had
routine cervical studies in a cancer survey project and
did not have previously diagnosed or treated cervical
cancer. Both groups were of similar economic status and
were patients of a charity hospital. The prevalence of
invasive carcinoma, intraepithelial carcinoma and
dysplasia was found to be higher in the Caucasian women
than in blacks. The remarkably higher relative
frequency of cervical cancer in blacks is not the result
of racial susceptibility but rather is associated with
factors relative to the lower socioeconomic status of
blacks in the United States.

486. Cobb, W. M. "The Negro Physician and Hospital Staffs,"
Hospital Management (March 1960):22-24.

A guest editorial which focuses on the contributions
made over the course of about 130 years in medicine by
black physicians. Acknowledging that progress has been
made in the equity of medical opportunities for blacks,
the author notes that only 2 percent of physicians in
the U.S. are black. With respect to hospital staffing,
the black physician has encountered the same obstacles
he once encountered by trying to enter into the medical
profession. Because of these barriers, many of the
physicians opened institutions around the country which
have served the needs of thousands of poor persons.

487. Cobb, W. M. "Integration in Medicine: A National
Need," Journal of the National Medical Association 49 (1)
(January 1957): 1-7.

Stresses the importance of integration in the medical
community to the health of blacks, makes specific
mention of the medical segregation found in Chicago and
praises the clarity of intention found in the name of
the Committee to End Discrimination in Chicago Medical
Institutions. The parallelism between this clarity of
name and the task of integrating the medical community
is the focus of the article. Describes early
developments of the black hospital concept and observes

that often times black patients were used for
experimental purposes and that many blacks died to
advance medical science. Also discusses the separate
facilities concept of black health care and notes that
the separate facilities concept often led to a "negro
medical ghetto." The negro physician became committed
to this separate and inferior system. Details the
weaknesses of the separate facilities system of negro
health care. Awareness of these weaknesses have led to
opposition to the segregated health care system.
Concludes by describing recent developments in the
struggle to end segregation in the medical community.

488. Condell, J. F. "The Negro Patient and Professional
Worker in the State-Supported Southern Mental Hospitals," The
Journal of Negro Education 23 (Spring 1954): 193-196.

In context of public policy of "separate but equal
facilities," investigates the extent of equality of
opportunity existing in the employment of black
professional workers in proportion to the number of
black patients in the state tax supported hospitals for
the mentally ill. Reports survey findings of mental
hospitals in 17 southern states. Finds that while
blacks represent an equal proportion of the mental
patients in state-supported mental hospitals to their
proportion the population of southern states, blacks are
not employed in the mental hospitals of four southern
states and in most professional categories in other
states. Only one state (Maryland) in the south employs
blacks in all four professional categories (M.D., RN,
MSW, Ph.D.).

489. Conn, Harold O. Sickle-Cell Trait and Splenic
Infarction Associated with High-Altitude Flying," The New
England Journal of Medicine 251 (11) (1954):417-420.

The author notes that until recently sickle cell trait
was not a contraindication to high altitude flying but
notes that recent reports indicate otherwise. Reports
on two cases and suggests that splenectomy, as reported
in earlier research, is not the treatment of choice
unless there are indications of the formation of an
abscess. Recommends that sickle cell testing of all
blacks on induction be performed and that positive
results be indicated on the records. These individuals
should then use surface transportation exclusively
during their military career. Emergency oxygen tanks
should be available on all military flights to allow
prophylactic oxygen to these men when aerial
transportation is mandatory.

490. Cooley, Jack C. "Clinical Triad of Massive Splenic
Infarction, Sicklemia Trait, and High Altitude Flying,"
Journal of the American Medical Association 154 (2) (January
9, 1954): 111-113.

Discusses the sicklemia trait with sudden splenic
enlargement following an airplane flight. The six cases

reported had a similar pattern. All six cases involved
blacks and their ages ranged from 23 years. All six
were examined after high altitude flying in
unpressurized aircraft of between 10,000 and 15,000
feet. Concludes that in five of the six, sickling was
demonstrated on laboratory preparation. Splenectomy is
the treatment that was chosen for all six cases. The
triad of sicklemia trait, high altitude flying, and
splenic infarction is discussed. Possible military
implications are mentioned.

491. Cornely, Paul. "Segregation and Discrimination in
Medical Care in the United States," American Journal of
Public Health 46 (September 1956):1074-81.

Addresses several issues including the lack of qualified
black health care professionals during the 1930's and
1940's. Group health insurance plans flourished during
the early 1930's, but this did not affect black health
care because no attempt was made to attract the black
segment of the population. Because of conditions in
World War II, a greater social consciousness emerged and
consequently black nurses and doctors were admitted to
various societies. Several recommendations for ending
health care discrimination include: 1) federal health
acts passed by Congress contain that nondiscriminatory
clauses and 2) state legislatures consider calling an
end to discriminatory practices.

492. Crump, E. Perry and Robinson, Judkin M. "Umbilical
Hernia: II. Occurrence in Negro Adolescents and Young
Adults," The Journal of Pediatrics 40 (6) (1952):777-780.

Umbilical hernias have been found to be higher in
infants and children among blacks than whites but they
usually close by age 4. The tendency to close has been
postulated but not studied in adolescents and young
adults. This study examined freshmen entering 3
Nashville institutions for umbilical hernias. Of 736
students, only 4 (0.5%) were found to have hernias. A
previous study of 382 Africans had found hernias in 6
percent of the cases, or 12 times the rate of the U.S.
study. A conclusion from the African study was that
there was a common hereditary factor in the African race
that predisposes to such hernias. Authors conclude that
the diluting influence of American racial admixture
reduced the incidence of umbilical hernia significantly
in the U.S.

493. Cunningham, Joseph A. and Hardenbergh, Firmon E.
"Comparative Incidence of Cholelithiasis in the Negro and
White Races," Archives of Internal Medicine 97 (1956): 68-72.

The purpose of this study was "to investigate the
overall incidence of cholelithiasis in Alabama and more
specifically to establish the comparative incidence of
this disease in the two races." The study was based on
6,185 consecutive autopsies performed in Alabama during
the period of 1946-1953. The results indicate that

cholelithiasis is found approximately four times as
frequently in the white race as in the black and that
the highest incidence is found in the white female
(11:125), the lowest in blacks. The findings clearly
show the roles of age in the disease - with, advancing
age, a steady rise in incidence is seen in the white
male and female. It is also noted in the black female
but is practically absent in the black male.

494. Cunningham, Robert M. "Negroes in Medicine: A
Breakthrough is Taking Place", The Modern Hospital 79 (2)
(August 1952): 67.

A brief editorial which examines the current-day status
(1952) of the black race in the field of medicine. Its
aim is to show that blacks are making a significant
breakthrough into medical field positions. The author
views this era as the beginning of sweeping changes in
the health care industry.

495. DeNatale, Albert, Caham, Amos, Jack, James, Race,
Robert and Sanger, Ruth "V. A 'New' Rh Antigen Common in
Negroes, Rare In White People." Journal of the American
Medical Association 159 (4) (September 24, 1955): 247-250.

Details the discovery of a "new" blood group antibody
exclusive to blacks and rare in whites, with the most
frequency being in New York blacks and West Africans.
The antibody was discovered in the serum of a white
patient (Mr. V.) who had received transfusions from 7
blacks. Addresses the issues of frequency, inheritance,
transfusion, and pregnancy. Concludes that V was indeed
a new antibody more common to blacks than whites. The
antigen was inherited as a dominant Mendelian character
and belonged to the Rh system. It had not been
determined, however, what its precise place in the Rh
system was.

496. Denney, William F., Finn, Thomas O. and Bird, Robert M.
"Clinical Diagnosis of Sickle-C Disease," Archives of
Internal Medicine 99 (1957): 214-217.

This report points to "the clinical differences between
sickle-cell anemia and sickle-c disease, which allow for
a diagnosis prior to laboratory identification of the
abnormal hemoglobin." The most important of these
abnormal hemoglobins are s- and c- hemoglobin. When the
two are present in the same person, a characteristic
syndrome may occur, which is designated as sickle-c
disease. Five cases of sickle-c disease in blacks are
described, and 41 previously reported cases are
reviewed. The data is contrasted with 16 cases of
electrophoretically proved sickle-cell anemia. "It is
felt that when a Negro patient with a positive
sickle-cell preparation has the findings of (1)
acthoragias, (2) abdominal cramps, (3) sphemomegaly, and
(4) more than 30 percent target cells in the peripheral
blood that an accurate clinical diagnosis of sickle-c
disease is possible."

497.   Derbes, Vincent J., Samuels, Monroe, Williams, Ollie
P., and Walsh, John J.   "Diffuse Leprosy: Case in a Louisiana
Negro," A.M.A. Archives of Dermatology 81 (January-June
1960):210-224.

    Describes a rarely seen case of Lucio phenomenon
leprosy. The black examined had never been outside the
State of Louisiana, yet displayed a form of leprosy that
Lucio in 1852 had determined was confined to Mexico.
The current patient was a 52 year old black male sawmill
worker from Alexandria, Louisiana who was admitted to
Charity Hospital in 1956. In 1951, the patient had
injured his legs with a saw. In the following years
infected lesions, recurring moderate pain, weight loss,
loss of eyebrows and eyelashes, anesthesia of
extremeties, and false-positive syphilis tests were
noted in the patient. Concludes that this black patient
was suffering from diffuse lepromatosis, and was the
first patient of non-Mexican ancestry to have been so
diagnosed.

498.   Dodson, Jack E., "The Differential Fertility Of The
Negro Population--Houston, Texas, 1940-1950, Milbank Memorial
Fund Quarterly 35 (3) (July 1957): 266-279.

    A discussion of the differential fertility of urban
black populations. Makes comparisons of changes in the
patterns of black and total white fertility from
1940-1950 in Houston, Texas. The comparisons of the
trends of change in black fertility involve: (1)
analysis of birth rates by age and birth order for the
total white and black women 15-44 years of age during
1940 and 1950, (2) analysis of birth rates by age and
birth order for the white and black married women 15-44
years of age during 1940 and 1950, (3) analysis of birth
rates for the Anglo-white, the Latin white, and the
black women for 1940 and 1950, (4) analysis of birth
and birth order rates by age for soicio-economic groups
of the black and Anglo-white populations for 1940 and
1950. Reports that black fertility tends to approximate
more closely the pattern of fertility of the white
population. There exists some evidence that color
differentials have diminished for urban populations in
recent years. The trend of the pattern of black
fertility for Houston from 1940 to 1950, however, does
not wholly support the hypothesis of converging
fertility patterns between color groups.

499.   Dummett, Clifton O.   "The Negro in Dental Education: A
Review of Important Occurrences," Phylon Quarterly 20
(December 1959): 379-388.

    The author traces the development of blacks in dental
education beginning with 1867. In that year, Harvard
University was the first university to establish a
dental school. Of its first six students, one was a
black. Despite the number of increasing black dentists,
he also mentions that the dentistry profession has not
been really popular with blacks and that few black

dentists had taken graduate education in dentistry.
Emphasizes developments at the dental schools of Howard
University and Meharry Medical College, since they have
been responsible for the education of the majority of
black dentists in the United States. Harlem Hospital
was the first predominantly black hospital to be
accredited by the American Dental Association.

500. Elgosin, Richard B., "Ingrown Hair in Beard," Journal
of The American Medical Association 151 (January-April
1953): 1156.

Discusses ingrown hairs in the neck area of blacks.
Suggests that blacks have curly hair that points to the
back of the skin. If allowed to grow, the hair
penetrates a nearby follicle. Once shaved, this sets up
an inflammatory reaction. The prevention is in daily
brushing and shaving the hairs, especially those on the
neck.

501. Erwin, Herbert J. "Psychiatric Medical Education Among
Negro Physicians," American Journal of Psychiatry 106
(February 1950): 624-627.

A historical discussion of the entrance of the black
race into the psychiatric field of study. Dr. Thomas P.
Brennan was the first black to do so in 1939. Discusses
the progress in general medical education and concludes
of the 199,733 living physicians, only 4,500 are blacks.
The widespread interest in psychiatric medical education
among blacks has been around only 10 years and that the
new and wider interest is being manifested by black
physicians by seeking training at the Graduate level.
Yet they are still lacking in placing research and
contributions to medical literature as a priority.

502. Ewing, Oscar R. "Facing the Facts of Negro Health,"
Crisis 59 (4) (April 1952):217-222, 261-262.

Discusses the health status of blacks in America and is
supportive of national health insurance which he
believes would make blacks financially capable of paying
for good health care. The author is Federal Security
Administrator. Argues that particular attention must be
paid to the health status of blacks. Although black
health has improved, "the average life expectancy at
birth of a white child is about sixty-eight years,
sixty-three years for Negro girls, and only little more
than fifty-eight years for Negro boys and twenty-nine
white babies die for every thousand live births, while
forty-seven Negro babies die for every thousand live
births." Concludes that national health insurance would
eliminate the economic inequality of the black patient.

503. Ferguson, A. D., Cutter, A. M. and Scott, R. B.
"Growth and Development of Negro Infants," The Journal of
Pediatrics 48 (1956): 308-313.

Analyzes certain environmental and cultural factors and determines the influence and relationship of these factors to the neuromotor development of black infants during the first year of life. The study focused on the development of 708 healthy, full-term black infants from various socioeconomic classes. Conclusions are drawn from data given in tables and bar graphs.

504. Fontanilla, Jose and Anderson, George. "Further Studies of the Racial Incidence and Mortality of Ectopic Pregnancy," American Journal of Obstetrics and Gynecology 70 (2) (August 1955):312-319.

Discusses the rate of ectopic gestations to live births for white women versus those of black women. The incidence of ectopic pregnancies was shown to be fifty percent higher in black women. The cause of this higher incidence of ectopic pregnancy was thought to be pelvic inflammatory disease, specifically gonorrhea. Over a period of five years, data showed that there was a decrease in the number of ectopic pregnancies in white women, yet the number in black women showed no change. Maternal deaths due to ectopic pregnancies were also higher in black women. However, quick diagnoses, more blood, and immediate surgery could have prevented some deaths in both black and white women. Concludes that the difference in incidences of ectopic pregnancies was due to the higher incidence of pelvic inflammatory disease in black women.

505. Frumkin, R. M. "Race and Major Mental Disorders," Journal of Negro Education 23 (Winter 1954): 97-98.

A study of first admissions to Ohio State Mental Hospitals for 1949 of blacks and whites. Finds that blacks had exceedingly higher rates of admission than whites and that the findings lend support to the hypothesis that there is a racial subgroup differential in the rates of first admissions which is inversely related to the factors of income, occupational prestige, education and socio-economic status. Concludes that the validity of the hypothesis is evidenced by higher rates of mental illness among blacks of low income, little education and low socio-economic status.

506. Galambos, John T. "Porphyria Cutanea Tarda Without Skin Lesion in an American Negro," American Journal of Medicine 25 (2) (August 1958): 315-320.

Porphyria cutanea tarda (PCT) without skin lesions is described in an American black. Large amounts of free porphyrins were present in the liver of this patient. He excreted greatly increased quantities of fecal porphyrins. The urine contained large quantities of uroporphyrins and increased amounts of coproporphyrins. No porphobilinogen was detectable on numerous examinations. The possible reasons for the absence of photosensitivity in this patient are discussed. There was no evidence of parenchymal liver disease until seven

years after the first signs of porphyria. It is
suggested that the underlying biochemical lesion caused
not only the abnormality in the porphyrin metabolism but
also could have been responsible for the subsequent
development of hepatocellular injury. There was no
demonstrable correlation in the diurnal excretion
patterns of urinary coproporphyrin (UCP) and urinary
uroporphyrin (UUP).

507. Garcia, Manuel. "The Curability of Carcinoma of the
Cervic in the Negro," Southern Medical Journal 45 (2)
(February 1952): 145-150.

   Discusses the high incidence of carcinoma of the cervix
   among colored women in the South and the difficulties
   associated with its treatment. Discusses radiation as
   the essential method of treatment in all the patients
   considered. Looks specifically at a case in Charity
   Hospital in New Orleans, Louisiana from April 1938 to
   the end of 1944. Points out that the survival rate
   among blacks is lower than whites; not because of their
   sensitivity to radiation; but because of the recognition
   of disease before treatment is sought. Concludes that
   radiation is effective in reoccurrence of the disease;
   specifically after five years of treatment of black
   cases.

508. Gelfand, H. M., LeBlance, D. R., Potash, L., Clemmer,
D. I. and Fox, J. P. "The Spread of Living Attenuated
Strains of Polioviruses in Two Communities in Southern
Louisiana," American Journal of Public Health 50 (6) (June
1960): 767-778.

   Living, attenuated poliovirus type 3 (Sabin vaccine) was
   administered orally early in June to all children in a
   group of families in two lower economic black
   communities in southern Louisiana which prior serologic
   study had shown to lack widespread natural immunity to
   this virus type. At the same time, in a group of
   similar families chosen to be the indicators of contact
   infection, a placebo material was fed. Study of
   frequent, routine fecal specimens from all children
   served to indicate primary and contact infections.
   Excretion of homologous virus occurred in 90 percent of
   vaccine-fed children during the succeeding seven weeks.
   Many concurrent "wild enterovirus infections" were
   detected. The failure of the vaccine strain to infect a
   larger proportion of the contact children was attributed
   in part to viral interference and in larger part to a
   lower infectiousness of the vaccine strain as compared
   with "wild" polioviruses.

509. Genovese, Eugene D. "Medical and Insurance Costs of
Slaveholding in the Cotton Belt." The Journal of Negro
History 45 (July 1960): 141-155.

   A survey of contemporaneous plantation and medical
   origins which establishes the significance of these
   terms to show a close relationship between economic and

medical history. A slave was an extreme annuity based
upon his predicted life-span and the estimated years of
productivity. Various kinds of epidemics were frequent
in the South and slaves losses occurred frequently.
Aside from the number of losses, it is relatively
impossible to evaluate the extent of the loss of a
particularly valuable slave. A portion of the insurance
cost would cover runaways. In St. Mary's Parish,
Louisiana, 100 slaves died and 400 others were taken
seriously ill from cholera. In Baton Rouge Parish from
June 1849 to June 1850, 143 slaves died from cholera.
John H. Randolph's papers estimate a slave valued at
$2,500 and was insured for $1,200 at 2.6 percent per
year. The cost of insuring slaves was undoubtedly much
higher than that for whites. Notes that two points must
be kept in mind when the figures are examined: few
planters kept books properly and much relevant data were
no doubt missing. Presents figures (estimations)
relative to the combined costs of medical attention,
insurance against premature death, and insurance against
runaways.

510. Giblett, Eloise R. and Chase, Jeanne. "Js a 'New'
Red-Cell Antigen Found in Negroes; Evidence for an Eleventh
Blood Group System," British Journal of Haemathology 5 (30)
(July 1959): 319-326.

The authors note the fact that the red cells of blacks
possess certain antigenic characteristics less common or
extremely rare in non-blacks. Describes a new blood
group antigen occurring in about 20 percent of blacks.
Evidence suggests that this antigen does not belong to
the ABO, MNS, Rh, Duffy, Kidd, or Diego systems, and
that it is probably not related to the Kell, P.,
Lutheran, or Lewis systems. Authors propose to name the
gene and its antigen "Sutter" in honor of the patient in
whom the corresponding antibody was discovered. In
1957, a young white male patient was given a blood
transfusion during an operation on his lung. One pint
of blood came from a black doctor. The patient
recovered uneventfully, but ten months later hemorrhaged
to death. Investigation of blood given to the patient
has led to the discovery and naming of a "new" red-cell
antigen.

511. Glaser, R. J. and Smith, D. E. (eds).
"Clinico-pathologic Conference: Aortic Aneurysm,
Hypertension, Heart Failure and Sudden Death," American
Journal of Medicine 12 (2) (February 1952): 244-259.

A clinical discussion was held at the Clinico-pathologic
Conference on the case of a black male, W. D. who was
admitted to the Barnes Hospital on August 8, 1950,
complaining of shortness of breath. The case is
reported in which disseminated histoplasmosis was
demonstrated in the patient who had typical clinical,
laboratory and biopsy findings of sarcoidosis.
Extensive study failed to establish whether the
histoplasmosis represented an invasion of pre-existent

sarcoidosis or whether the histoplasmosis was responsible for the granulomatous lesions which simulated sarcoidosis. The diagnosis of sarcoidosis should be made only by exclusion. Tuberculosis and granulomatosis as well as histoplasmosis may simulate sarcoidosis and must be excluded by appropriate studies before the diagnosis of sarcoidosis is warranted.

512. Gleich, M., Smoller, S., and Scott, B. E. "Calcium and Phosphorus Studies in Negro Premature Infants," The Journal of Pediatrics 39 (6) (1951):677-679.

The authors observe that premature infants are very susceptible to rickets. They undertook chemical studies of premature infants at the Pediatric Service of Harlem Hospital of New York City. Prior to discharge, they placed the infants on a milk formula diet and on high potency multivitamins. There was no evidence of rickets biochemically or roentgenographically in the group. They concluded that "a simple half-skim milk or evaporated milk formula supplemented with 1,000 U.S.P. units of vitamin D daily prevented the development of rickets in these premature infants up to the time of discharge.

513. Goldstein, Marcus S. "Longevity and the Health Status of the Negro American," The Journal of Negro Education 32 (Fall 1959): 337-348.

A discussion of the major changes in the health status of the nonwhite segment (mainly blacks) of the American population during this decade. Focuses on longevity, rates of mortality, morbidity (including mental illness), and availability of medical care. Argues that blacks would survive in the U.S. mainly because of their high fertility rate. According to the author, black birth rates were 30 percent higher than white birth rates. Despite the serious health problems confronting blacks, they will survive a long time, not because of improving health, but because there large numbers.

514. Goldstein, Rhoda L. "Negro Nurses in Hospitals," American Journal of Nursing 60 (February 1960):215-217.

A study of black nurses on the nursing staffs of several hospitals. Notes that the extreme nursing shortage during World War II led, with much resignation, to the hiring of black nurses in many all white hospitals. In determining the experiences of the black nurses, the nature of the hospital as an institution and the nurse's role in the hospital played large roles. The largest obstacle for the black nurse involves acceptance on the part of both her colleagues and patients.

515. Grant, Faye and Groom, Dale. "A Dietary Study Among a Group of Southern Negroes," Journal of the American Dietetic Association 35 (September 1959):910-918.

A study of the effects of dietary habits of Southern
blacks and the effects of their eating habits on their
health in Charleston, South Carolina. The study
consisted of visiting 59 families over a period of four
weeks. The findings were surprising since most of the
families exhibited a passable balanced diet. A
plausible explanation for the unexpected results is due
to the fact that many of the people interviewed lived on
or near farms, thereby providing access to a variety of
fresh fruits and vegetables found on many of the farms.

516. Greene, Charles R. and Kelly, John J.
"Electrocardiogram of the Healthy Adult Negro," Circulation
20 (November 1959): 206-209.

The "T" waves of precordial electrocardiograms are
upright in healthy adult white subjects. In contrast,
reports have drawn attention to "T" wave inversion
"juvenile pattern" in adult blacks free of organic heart
disease. This study could detect no increased incidence
of the "juvenile pattern" in healthy adult blacks. The
authors note an identical standard for normality for
both whites and blacks. Any abnormalities will have to
be explained as caused by a source other than that of
race. Data was drawn from 144 healthy blacks (105
females and 39 males) varying in age from 18 to 69. The
group was composed of hospital employees, nurses, and
resident physicians, and most were native or long-term
residents of New York. None had a history of inadequate
diet. In summation, the electrocardiograms for the
entire group were within the normal range.

517. Groom, Dale. "A Comparative Study of Coronary Disease
in Haitian and American Negroes," Southern Medical Journal 52
(May 1959): 504-510.

Discusses the pathologic evaluation of coronary and
aortic atherosclerosis in 267 autopsies of blacks and
Haitians. Notes almost double the degree of coronary
disease among the American blacks. This held true for
both males and females at all age decades over twenty.
Concludes that prominent environmental differences in
these two populations include those of stress, tempo,
physical exertion and competiveness, in addition to
diet. Suggests that factors other than diet affect the
incidences of coronary disease in blacks and Haitians.

518. Grossack, M. "Psychology in Negro Colleges," American
Psychologist 98 (October 1954): 636-637.

A report of a mail survey to determine characteristics
of psychology programs in black colleges. Finds
exceptionally low ratio of Ph.D. instructors to
non-Ph.D. instructors in black colleges. Concludes that
faculties in black colleges are less competent than
faculties in non-black colleges, that a "major" in
psychology is not offered in vast majority of black
colleges and that the lack of competent faculties and

undergraduate majors indicates need for professional attention to develop programs in black colleges.

519.   Hammer, Emanuel F.   "Frustration-Aggression Hypothesis Extended to Socio-Racial Areas: Comparison of Negro and White Children's H-T-P's," Psychiatric Quarterly 27 (October 1953):597-607.

Extends the hypothesis that while economic discrimination against blacks may or may not represent rejection, social discrimination against blacks must, almost by definition in our culture, represent rejection and, hence, eventuate in frustration. The black child feels the reflected differences in opportunity hand the comparatively meager advantages that are presented to his parents, as opposed to the greater opportunities and advantages presented to the parents of his white contemporaries. The test used to validate the hypothesis consisted of allowing black children to draw, free-hand, a house, a tree and a person (HTP). For black children, as compared to whites, the drawings represented a mean hostility rating of almost triple that of the white children.

520.   Henington, V. Medd, Kennedy, C. Barrett, and Snider, Kenneth B.   "Bullous Dermatoses in the Southern Negro," Southern Medical Journal 49 1 (January 1956):39-46.

Discusses various skin diseases (bullous dermatoses) found in 105 blacks over a five year period and the differentiation of severity between blacks and whites. One factual difference discussed was the general poor health of blacks and the role this played in making him less prone to recovery from dermatoses. Also, blacks were known to have complete lack of resistance to pustular types of skin dermatitis and it was usually not diagnosed until the secondary state. Bullous dermatoses were more frequent in blacks than in whites and more serious (7 deaths out of the 105 cases). Points out the nine types of bullous dermatoses found along with the number of cases of each, how each was handled, and the outcome. One category discussed was drug eruptions and under that category fell 33 cases of which 17 were caused by indiscriminate consumption of the medicine "666." Most patients refuse to stop taking the medication and recurrences were frequent. Concludes that differences in skin diseases between whites and blacks did exist but the racial differentiation should not be taken too far.

521.   Herrera, J. M.   "Sickle Cell Anemia and Pulmonary Tuberculosis," Journal of the American Medical Association 146 (3) (May 19, 1951): 292-293.

A study of sickle cell anemia in a group of 138 adolescence. The investigation showed the presence of sickle cell in 8 out of the 138. Two had sickle cell anemia. Six including the two had pulmonary tuberculosis. Discusses current treatment and how it

has failed. Concludes that sickle cell aggravates
pulmonary tuberculosis and that the course of the
disease is more acute in blacks and Mulattoes.

522. Hilliard, George W. "Meigs' Syndrome: A Report of a
Case," Journal of the American Medical Association 151 (9)
(February 28, 1953): 738-740.

   Describes a case of Meigs' syndrome in a black. The
   patient was a 57 year old woman whose primary complaints
   were abdominal enlargement, dyspeq, and abdominal pain.
   The criteria of Meigs' syndrome, the presence of an
   ovarian fibroma with ascites and pleural fussion, are
   fulfilled in the case. Discusses the history of the
   disease and its introduction to the medical field in
   1932 by five reported cases. Concludes that the disease
   usually occurs in women past menopause. The symptoms of
   the disease may run from days to years.

523. Hockwald, Robert S. "Toxicity of Primaquine in
Negroes," Journal of the American Medical Association 149 (1)
(August 23, 1952): 1568-1570.

   A study of Primaquine in blacks. Concludes that doses
   of 30 milligrams of base is too toxic if used in blacks
   without close medical supervision. The study used 110
   black volunteers to test the drug and discovered 5
   percent contracted severe progressive anemia. The
   anemia was of the same magnitude as that developing
   after the administration of pamaquine, 30 milligrams
   base daily. Concludes that primaquine 15 milligrams of
   base can be given safely to adult blacks for 14 days
   without special medical supervision.

524. Holly, Pearl B., Felts, Jr., William R. and Rheingold,
Jack J. "Pernicious Anemia Occuring Simultaneously in
Identical Negro Twins," A.M.A. Archives of Internal Medicine
90 (1952): 707-710.

   A case report of the simultaneous occurrence of
   pernicious anemia in 72 year old identical female black
   twins. The twins developed anemia within a few weeks of
   each other. Each member of the twins was admitted to
   the hospital for proper diagnosis and treatment.
   Improvement was noticed and continued after discharge
   from the hospital. After discharged from the hospital,
   the twins continued on the same diet and remained well.
   It was noted that the cause of the disease was not from
   nutritional deficiency. The article concluded that the
   genetic implications of the disease was that the
   evidence points to the monozygocity of the twins.

525. Irby, R., Hennigar, G. R. and Kirk, J. "Acute
Disseminated Lupus Erythematus in the Negro Male: Report of
Case with Autopsy Findings," Annals of Internal Medicine 37
(1952): 1274-1280.

   Reports the first case of acute disseminated lupus
   erythematosus in the oldest black male recorded. The

case report provides a lengthy synopsis of the patient's
initial reporting, physical examination, laboratory
results, hospital stay, and autopsy after death.
Attention was called to the unusual massive involvement
of the lymph glands and the pericarditis which was
determined to be the probable cause of death.

526.   Irby, R.   "Congenital Hemolytic Anemia in Negro
Brothers," Journal of the American Medical Association 153
(2) (1953):103-104.

Congenital hemolytic anemia in blacks was a rare entity
until 1944. However, it has become apparent that the
disease in blacks is recognized more frequently.
Because the disease may be benign in itself, splenectomy
has been refused in many cases in the past. Only 4 of
the 18 previously reported patients were black men.
After the diagnosis of congenital hemolytic anemia was
made in the two patients, splenectomy was performed in
both and was followed by the disappearance of evidence
of increased hemolysis and reticulocytosis, although
microspherocytosis and increased fragility remained.
The mother of the patients was found to have no evidence
of jaundice, splenomegaly, or anemia.

527.   James, Milton M.   "Comparative Mental Abilities of
Negroes and Whites," The Negro History Bulletin 15 (April
1952):137-141.

Focuses on the research that has attempted to show the
difference between white and black mental abilities.
Argues that the differences in intelligence are due to
the differences in educational opportunities which may
affect both the physical and mental development of the
child. In fact, many black children do better than the
average white child in spite of all the handicaps to
which the former has been subjected. The conclusion is
inescapable that any decision to use differences in the
average achievement of the two racial groups as a basis
for classifying in advance any child, negro or white, is
scientifically unjustified.

528.   Jenkins, Melvin E., Scott, Roland B. and Baird, Robert
L.   "Studies in Sickle Cell Anemia," The Journal of
Pediatrics 56 (1) (January 1960): 30-38.

The authors review a study of ten sickle cell anemia
cases in order to explain the occurrence of sudden death
in those persons afflicted with the disease. The
authors note that such instances of sudden death while
relatively rare, yet are quite perplexing. Observe that
instances of sudden death "associated with splenic
engangement and infarction have been reported in Negro
soldiers with sickle cell trait during airplane flights
at high altitude." The authors propose a possible
explanation: a mechanism of stasis of red blood cells in
the spleen, liver, or splanchnic capallaries when
combined with vascular collapse and cerebral anoxia.
The authors believe this condition would explain the

sudden death of black infants already debilitated by
anemia, hemolysis and infection.

529. Johnson, Joseph L. "Opportunities for Negroes in
Undergraduate Medical Education in 1952," Journal of the
National Medical Association 44 (5) (September 1952):
353-355.

    A concern about improving opportunities for blacks to
secure adequate medical education and presents data from
1947-1952 of the number of medical schools with blacks
enrolled. Notes an increase of only 20 schools over a
five year period. Also lists the medical schools with
the most black students: Meharry Medical College and
Howard University. Concludes that to assure continued
increase of opportunities for blacks in undergraduate
medical education there must be a very marked
strengthening of the preparation of black students at
the elementary, secondary and college levels. There
must be a larger number of black students who can
successfully compete on the basis of preparation for
admission to all medical schools.

530. Kahle, H. R., Jackson, J. T. "Cholecystitis in Negro
Children," Journal of the American Medical Association 151
(15) (1953):1269-1271.

    Two cases of Cholecystitis, one subacute and the other
acute suppurative, are reported in black children. The
disease is uncommon in childhood and is much less
frequent in blacks than in whites at all periods of
life. Etiology, diagnosis, and management are briefly
discussed.

531. Kahn, Jane and Gildea, Margaret C. L. "Group Therapy
for Parents of Behavior Problem Children in Public Schools,"
American Journal of Psychiatry 108 (July 1951):351-356.

    Explores the failure of a group therapy project for
parents of behavior problem children in public schools
in black areas. Explanations for the failure lay in
minority tensions and anxieties between group members
which made it impossible for the black mothers to face
responsibility for their children. The problems of
their children could not be felt by them as clear cut
issues without contamination by ideas of discrimination.
Another explanation for the failure of the project was
the low educational-cultural level of the black
population.

532. Keller, D. H. and Johnson, J. B. "The T Wave of the
Unipolar Precordial Electrocardiogram in Normal Adult Negro
Subjects," American Heart Journal 44 (4) (October 1952):
494-498.

    Appears that the T wave in precordial electrocardiograms
of normal black adult subjects may be inverted over the
right precordium extending as far as the left sternal
line. Persistence of T-wave inversion farther to the

left is generally considered abnormal. In contrast,
others have reported T-wave inversion over the left
precordium as far as the left midclavicular line in
Mexican, black, and Puerto Rican adults who were said to
be normal subjects. A study of the T-wave in unipolar
precordial electrocardiograms of eighty-five nornal
adult black subjects has been presented which confirms
the standard generally accepted for normal adults. In
this series of normal adults, no instance of T-wave
inversion was found in the left or the V_2 position, and
in only one instance was an inverted T wave found in V_2.

533. Kennedy, Janet A. "Problems Posed in the Analysis of
Negro Patients," Psychiatry 15 (30) (August 1952): 313-327.

Two problem areas of difference exist between black and
white patients in seeking psychiatric treatment. First,
black patients usually enter treatment with fear,
suspicion and distrust regardless of whether the
therapist is black or white. Second, the ego in a black
is "blurred by the phenomenon of color." Two black
women were selected in the therapy to show how
particular fate of the black in-group affects the result
to the therapy. One patient showed improvement in the
process from her behavior patterns while the other
failed. The patients who failed in the therapy could
not faced the unrealistic character of her white ego
ideal. The social aspect also plays a part in blacks as
they grow up. Such as the advertising was usually
addressed to the urban black that the "white way is the
right way." Products like skin bleacher and hair
straightener often appeared in most of the
advertisements. The special burdens of therapy imposed
upon of black patients are (1) the white stereotype of
the therapist and the black stereotype of the patient
and (2) the aspiration level of the patients.

534. Kirchoff, Helen. "Frequency of Cancer in the White and
Negro," Southern Medical Journal 49 (August 1956): 834-841.

Discusses the history of cancer and notes that the
incidence of malignant cancer among blacks is much less
than whites. Discusses the following points: (1) the
percentage of tumors found in the gastrointestinal tract
is the same for the male in both races; (2) there is no
significant difference in the percentage of tumors found
in the gastrointestinal tract in the white and black
female; (3) cancer of the breast is more frequent among
the cancer cases found in the black female than in the
white female; and (4) cancer of the genital tract is
statistically more frequent in the black than in the
white. Reports on the frequency of cancer in the
autopsies performed between 1920 and 1954 in the John
Sealy Hospital and argues that cancer occurs more
frequently in the white than the black.

535. Kirschenfeld, J. J. "Prevalence and Significance of
Anemia as Seen in a Rural General Practice," Journal of the
American Medical Association 158 (1) (July 9, 1955): 807-810.

Discusses Anemia in blacks in Alabama and its
relationship to blacks as a whole. Presents data on the
incidences of Anemia to be about 10 to 15 percent in the
white race and 20 to 25 percent in blacks. The chief
cause of Anemia in blacks is poor diet, excessive blood
loss, or combinations. Notes that 39 percent of the
cases of blacks with Anemia was a result of iron
deficiency. Discusses different treatments and cures
for the disease including a proper diet, iron salt
regulation, the source of infection and the loss of
blood.

536. Kiser, Clyde V. "Fertility And Differentials Among
Nonwhites In The United States." Milbank Memorial Fund
Quarterly 36 (2) (April 1958): 149-196.

Examines trends and differentials in the fertility of
nonwhites in the United States but deals primarily with
blacks. Graphs and tables are presented which show the
birth and death rates per 1,000 population by color in
the United States from 1915-1955. Points out that
nearly 16 million people were enumerated as nonwhites in
the 1950 Census of the United States. Nearly 96 percent
of these were blacks. During 1940-1955, the crude birth
rate increased by 28 percent whites and by 30 percent
for nonwhites. Notes that much of the increase in
fertility of young nonwhites was due to a remarkable
decline of childlessness. Attributes the decrease of
childlessness among blacks in the U.S. as having
occurred during a period of medical discoveries and
community action for reduction of venereal disease.
They occurred in the context of advance in the economic,
educational and civic status of blacks in the United
States.

537. Laufman, Harold. "Profound Accidental Hypothermia,"
Journal of the American Medical Association 147 (13)
(November 24, 1951): 1201-1207.

Reports on a severe case of Hypothermia in a black woman
age 23. She had been found in an alley in a frozen
coma. Discusses her temperature recovery curve, blood
chemistry, hematologic findings, results of urinalysis,
and electrocardiogram. Observes that the critical level
in humans for hypothermia is between 68-74 degrees. The
woman was below the 68 degree mark.

538. Lee, Everett S. and Lee, Anne S. "The Differential
Fertility of the American Negro," American Sociological
Review 17 (August 1952): 434-437.

The authors feature several charts which explain
fertility rates of blacks under various circumstances.
Notes that fertility rates for blacks are higher in
rural areas than urban areas, and inside the South than
outside it. The socioeconomic backgrounds seem to play
a major role here. The tables relate fertility ratios
to such variables as place of residence, employment
status, tenure of home, monthly rental value of home,

and number of school years completed. In addition, the
tables examine the relationship of variables to each
other such as rural versus urban residence, and the
marital status of the mother. Concludes that more
favorable socioeconomic status affects the decline of
fertility for both blacks and whites.

539. Lindau, Warren. "Subacute Disseminated Lupus
Erythematosus in the Negro Male," Southern Medical Journal 46
(11) (November 1953): 1099-1102.

Discusses Lupus Erthematosus in the black male. Up to
the time, only four cases had been reported. The
occurrence of a fifth case in a black male resulted in
the study being done. Presents a case report on the
male who was 33 years old, a postal clerk, and was
hospitalized after three days of fever and chills. The
male died and an autopsy was performed that found the
characteristic symptoms of the disease. Notes that this
is the first case of subacute form to be reported in a
black male.

540. Love, W. D. and Burch, G. "Plasma and Erythrocyte
Sodium and Potassium Concentrations in a Group of Southern
White and Negro Blood Donors," Journal of Laboratory and
Clinical Medicine 41 (1953): 258-267.

A study of 62 male and 43 female subjects from 18 to 60
years of age (48 whites and 57 blacks) at Charity
Hospital in New Orleans. Describes the methodology of
collecting blood samples, centrifugation and analysis
for sodium and potassium. Experimental error is
discussed for chemical determination of plasma and red
blood cells. The authors offer three extensive tables
of statistical data and results. Also included is a
brief discussion of the effect on the study of including
blacks with sickle-cell disease and of the effect of the
trait on the concentration of red cell sodium.

541. Malzberg, Benjamin. "Marital Status and Mental Disease
Among Negroes in New York State," The Journal of Nervous and
Mental Disease 128 (January 1956): 457-463.

A study of the relative distribution of mental disease
according to marital status based upon average annual
rates of the first admissions among blacks to all
hospitals for mental disease in New York State from July
1, 1938 to June 30, 1941. Previous studies had shown
that there are marked differences in such rates, the
single (unmarried) having rates substantially higher
than those for the married. This is due in part to the
action of marriage, which selects the more stable and
healthy and leaves the unstable within the ranks of the
unmarried.

542. Malzberg, Benjamin. "Use of Alcohol Among White and
Negro Mental Patients," Quarterly Journal on Studies on
Alcohol 16 (1955):668-74.

Discusses the frequency of alcoholic psychoses among blacks first admissions to hospitals for mental disease in the state of New York. Argues that excessive drinking may play a significant role in the frequency of these psychoses. Concludes that black first admissions have higher rates of these psychoses than white first admissions.

543. McIntosh, H. N. "Dental Hypoplasais in Congenital Syphilis," Journal of the American Medical Association 146 (11) (July 14, 1951): 1075-1076.

A report of a survey of 18 public schools for blacks in Missouri to determine the incidence of congenital syphilis in children with dental hypoplasais suggestive of syphilis. The public health dentist examined 1,639 children. The family of each seropositive child was examined by the medical officers. Of the 54 that were examined, 50 were tested for syphilis and 16 were found to be infected with congenital syphilis. Results concluded that the cooperation of dentists would be of practical value in case findings; and findings could expect to show 25 percent of the patients infected with congenital syphilis.

544. McLean, Franklin, Reitzes, Hilda, and Calloway, N. O. "Progress in Chicago," Modern Hospital 79 (August 1952):68-70.

A sample study of Chicago to determine if the barriers of segregation were breaking down with regards to blacks being on medical staffs of hospitals, students in unsegregated medical schools, and having positions on faculties. Upon receipt of a number of questionnaires, the authors found that progress was being made. Before World War II, only a few hospitals in the U.S. had both white and black physicians working together. By 1951, there was a 400 percent increase in the number of blacks becoming physicians. But the authors are careful to point out that although the quality of education provided to blacks in the area of medicine has improved substantially, the proportion of black physicians to the black community had remained unchanged.

545. McLoughlin, Christopher J., Petrie, Lester M., and Hodgins, Thomas E. "Diagnostic Significance of Blood Sugar Findings." Journal of the American Medical Association 153 (September-December 1953): 182-184.

Demonstrates in Georgia an effective procedure for screening large cross sections of the population on a voluntary basis using the Anthrone method of blood sugar analysis. Finds that a definite higher prevalence of abnormal carbohydrate metabolism exists in the black woman and that the incidence gets higher in the older age group. Suggests that an educational program be developed in the state of Georgia to bring physicians up-to-date on modern usage of diagnostic criteria of this disease.

546. McVay, Leon V., Jr., and Keil, Philip G. "Myocardial Infarction with Special Reference to the Negro," _Archives of Internal Medicine_ 96 (1955): 762-767.

>   Compares salient features of coronary artery disease in white and black patients. In the study of 330 cases, the incidence of mycordial infarction in blacks was found to be only 42 percent of that in white patients. Myocardial infarction occurs earlier in the black woman than in the black man, white man, or white woman and is equally frequent among black men and women, while among the white patients it was three times as common among the men. Concludes that further investigation of coronary atherosclerosis and myocardial infarction in the black women is necessary.

547. Meredith, H. V. "North American Negro Infants: Size at Birth and Growth During First Postnatal Year," _Human Biology_ 24 (1952): 290-308.

>   Discusses two generalizations pertaining to North American black neonates: (1) the birth weight of blacks is smaller than that of whites, and (2) blacks in favorable social and economic conditions tend to be comparable to whites at birth. The article is divided into a discussion on size at birth up to the eighth postnatal week and a second discussion on growth during the first year of infancy which focuses on four successive quarter-year ages, from 3 months to 1 year. Tables give comparative periodic data for black and white babies as published in the literature of the era.

548. Mullin, Frederick, Cunningham, Robert M., and Anderson, Donald. "Round Table on Current Problems," _The Modern Hospital_ 79 (2) (August 1952): 74-75, 134.

>   A summary of a roundtable seminar discussion on the progress that the black race has made in recent years in entering the health care industry as part of its working force.

549. Myerson, R. M., Harrison, E. and Lohmuller, H. W. "Incidence and Significance of Abnormal Hemoglobins: Reports of a Series of 1,000 Hospitalized Negro Veterans," _American Journal of Medicine_ 26 (4) (April 1959): 543-546.

>   Hemoglobin electrophoresis was performed in blood samples of 1,000 consecutive hospitalized black veterans. Abnormalities were detected in 10.6 percent, a figure comparable to that of other large series. The abnormalities included seventy-four patients with AS hemoglobin, twenty-three with AC, three with SS, two with SC and one with AD. Three patients had increased amounts of F hemoglobin. A survey of the clinical records of these patients revealed three instance of gross hematuria in the AS group, one in the AC group and one in the SC group. Nephrectomy had been performed on two of these five patients. One patient with SC disease was asymptomatic and the only abnormality in the

fifty-seven year old man with SS hemoglobin was a
moderate anemia. This study re-emphasizes the potential
clinical and genetic importance of the
hemoglobinopathies and questions the supposed benignancy
of the trait patterns.

550. "Negro in Florida." Time 59 (January 14, 1952):
71-72.

Dr. George Henry Starke, a young black doctor, fresh
from Meharry Medical College, learned what it was all
about to be a black doctor in the heart of Florida's
orange-grove country. He started practicing at a time
when he had to turn his patients over to white doctors
because they felt that he was not able to make a correct
diagnosis. After 24 years of practicing Dr. Starke
opened a $50,000 clinic and established a solid record
for helping to find a successful treatment for pneumonia
by using sulfa drugs.

551. "The Negro Health Crusade Goes On." Hygiene (May,
1951): 330-331.

Several black organizations have sponsored activities to
improve the health of blacks. One such activity is
Negro Health Week which is sponsored during the first
week in April. Also celebrated at this time is the
birthday of Booker T. Washington who originated the
institution of Negro Health Week in 1915. Dr.
Washington is also credited for revealing startling
facts concerning the health of the colored people of the
United States. It was shown that 45 per cent of all the
deaths among blacks were preventable and about 450,000
blacks were seriously ill all the time. It was
estimated that the life expectancy in the American black
is shorter by ten years than in the white man.

552. "Negroes' Contribution to Science and Invention." The
Negro History Bulletin 18 (April 1955): 153.

Points out contributions of several blacks to medical
science. Daniel Hale Williams, born in 1858, proved to
be a good counselor and friend to his patients. His
services were so tremendous that he became a member of
the Illinois State Board of Health. Dr. Williams was
credited with performing the first successful surgical
closure of a wound of the heart. Another great was Dr.
William A. Hinton, bacteriologist, who was credited for
developing a test for determining the presence of
syphilis. The test was used by the U.S. Public Health
Service. Dr. Carles Drew, world authority in blood
substitutes, was instrumental in saving countless number
of lives with blood plasma projects in World War II.
These men have all come in contact with prejudice and
discrimination, but have not let these obstacles prevent
them from contributing their talents to society.

553. "Negroes in the Professions," Journal of Negro History
43 (July 1958): 196-198.

Presents data and information regarding blacks in the medical profession. In 1891, there were 27 black doctors and 4 black lawyers in the state of Georgia. By 1900, there were 43 doctors, 14 lawyers and 10 dentists. Most of these doctors were located in only 28 counties, which meant that most of the blacks residing in rural areas were dependent upon white doctors, or had no medical services available to them. Dr. R. D. Badger of Atlanta, after receiving his freedom from his owner located his successful dental practice on fashionable Peachtree. However, protests from white citizens caused the Atlanta City Council to pass an ordinance prohibiting blacks from practicing in the profession in 1859. After the war, Dr. Badger established a lucrative practice in 1890 and acquired a $9,600 estate. Dr. Simeon Palmer Lloyd of Savannah, Georgia, was the first black to be appointed as one of the four city physicians in 1894 by Mayor Meyer and his council. Dr. Lloyd was the son of Josiah D. Lloyd, a successful grocerman and the oldest black citizen in business during that time. Dr. Lloyd graduated with distinctions from Atlanta University in 1869 and entered the medical department of the University of Pennsylvania where he graduated with honors in May, 1893. At the end of his first year as a physician, Dr. Lloyd reported that he had treated 6,712 black patients and 224 whites.

554. "Negroes Resist Malaria," Science News Letter 68 (July 23, 1955):52.

A team of United States Public Health Service scientists finds that blacks are highly resistant to the common malaria of the United States in comparison to whites. In the course of treatment of syphilis, 104 black and 529 white patients were inoculated with the parasite that causes benign tertian malaria. Almost ninety seven percent of the whites contracted the infection, while only 23.1 percent of the blacks became ill. During the test, one black received an inoculation containing over one billion parasites. This patient showed no parasites in his blood the following day or thereafter. In contrast, whites receiving only one-tenth this number often showed parasites in their blood immediately, and they may be present continuously throughout the primary attack.

555. Olansky, Sidney, Harris, Ad, Cutler, John C., and Price, Eleanor V. "Untreated Syphilis in the Male Negro," Archives of Dermatology 73 (May 1956):516-529.

Details a twenty-two year study of 431 syphilitic men. Of these 431 men, 176 men (40.8 percent) died by the end of the study. The death rate ranged from 18 percent for those with syphilis of ten years or less (at the time of admission to the study) to 96 percent among those who had syphilis 40 years or more at the time of admission to the study. Points out various tests given throughout the duration of the study and the reactions (positive, negative, etc.) to these tests. Tables show various

data dealing with the duration of the infection as
related to the death rate and the status of the patients
at the end of the study.

556. Olansky, Sidney, Schuman, Stanley, Peters, Jesse,
Smith, C. A., and Rambo, Dorothy S. "Untreated Syphilis in
the Negro Male," Journal of Chronic Disease 4 (2) (August
1956):177-185.

Details observations of 600 patients in the Tuskegee
syphilis study. This group included those with
untreated syphilis and some that were presumed to be non
syphilitic. Special attention was given to evidence of
late syphilis and abnormalities of the cardiovascular
system in both groups. The study showed that there was
a higher rate of cardiac problems in the syphilitic
group which caused the doctors to suggest that syphilis
could predispose a patient to heart problems. Also more
common in the syphilitic group was blood pressure
abnormalities. Concludes that problems with diagnosing
syphilis in the aged were complex and often involved the
cardiovascular system.

557. Pariser, Harry. "Treatment of Blastomycosis with
Stilbamidine," Journal of the American Medical Association
152 (14) (May 9, 1952): 129-131.

A case report of a 53 year old black man with systemic
blastomycosis. Points out that the disease is
relatively uncommon, but frequently fatal where there is
no satisfactory treatment available. Discusses a drug
called Stilbamidine and reports its success on the case
of the man. The drug was given for 29 days and all
cutaneous lesions and systemic symptoms of blastomycosis
disappeared following the therapy.

558. Payton, Eleanor, Crump, E. Perry and Horton, Carrell P.
"Growth and Development," Journal of the American Dietetic
Association 37 (August 1960):129-136.

The dietary records of 571 pregnant black women are
calculated and assessed in terms of nutritional
allowances recommended during pregnancy. In comparing
the level of recommended nutrients, only one vitamin was
found to be in conjunction with the recommendations for
pregnant women. Economic circumstances, food dislikes,
and often times, an obvious lack of knowledge concerning
nutritional needs, explain the reasons for the omissions
concerning the nutrients.

559. Pennell, Maryland and Grover, Mary. "Urban and Rural
Mortality From Selected Causes in the North and South,"
Public Health Reports 66 (10) (March 9, 1951):295-305.

A detail analysis of the seven leading causes of death
among blacks and the margin by which they exceeded the
death rates of the white population. The seven causes
of death included tuberculosis, nephritis, influenza and
pneumonia, intracranial lesions of vascular origins,

diseases of the heart, syphilis, and homicide. Tables
are used to indicate the number of non-white deaths in
the North versus the South as well as the tendency of
each disease in areas of various population sizes. The
conclusion notes that homicide has the greatest tendency
in the non-white population and suicide has the greatest
tendency in the white population.

560. Pennell, Maryland and Lehman, Josephine. "Mortality
From Heart Disease Among Negroes as Compared with White
Persons," Public Health Reports 66 (3) (January 9,
1951):57-75.

Compares heart mortality of blacks and whites in
relation to the effect of differences in environment in
urban and rural parts of the several geographic sections
of the United States with special attention to sex and
age. The distribution of the populations studied is
listed along with the types of heart diseases. Various
graphs are used to illustrate the comparisons between
males-females as well as variations in age and color as
well as population-size differences. Concludes that
black heart mortality is higher in the North than in the
South, higher in urban than in rural areas, higher in
males than in females, and higher in the young than in
the old. Black mortality curves for six of the eight
forms of heart disease are higher than the white curves
for almost every age group.

561. Perlman, L. P., Berstein, A., Maslow, W. C., and
Scatliff, J. H. "Gout in a Negro Woman," Journal of the
American Medical Association 151 (9) (1953):727-728.

A report of Gout in a 50 year old black woman, a disease
which had been rarely reported in black women. In this
case, the black woman met all the diagnostic criteria.
Initial episode of pain occurred in right big toe and
moved to the knees, elbows, wrists, and hands within one
year. Pictures, lab results and X-rays are presented.
There are only 5 perviously reported cases of Gout in
blacks.

562. Poore, John B., Mermann, Alan and Yu, Julia S.
"Adrenal-Cortical Carcinoma and Melanocarcinoma in a 5-Year
Old Negro Child," Cancer 7 (Summer 1955):1235-1241.

Discusses the case of a 5 year old black boy who has an
androgenic adrenalcotical carcinoma and a
melanocarcinoma of the buccal mucosa. No such case has
ever been reported. Among the unusual features of the
case was an unexpected regression of the buccal-mucosal
melanocarcinoma following hormone therapy. Such a
response warrents further study.

563. Portnoy, B. and Chalmer, L. S. "A Comparative Study of
Negro and White Subnormals on the Children's Form of the
Rosenzweig P-F Test," American Journal of Mental Deficiency
59 (2) (October 1954): 272-278.

Thirty institutionalized subnormal white children (15 males; 15 females) and 30 institutionalized black children (15 males; 15 females) were tested with the Children's Form of the Rosenzweig Picture-Frustration Test. The males and females in both groups were matched for chronological age, mental age, intelligence quotient, and length of institutionalization. The performance of the white and black subnormal groups were compared with one another with Rosenzweig's normative group. It was shown that the black and total (black plus white) subnormal groups were more Impunitive than the normal group; the normal groups was more Ego-Defensive than the white. Black and total groups of subnormals, and the black, white and total groups were more Need-Persistent than the normal group.

564. Postell, William D. "Birth and Mortality Rates Among Slave Infants on Southern Plantations," _Pediatrics_ 10 (November 1952):538-541.

Discusses the health care of the slave infants in the Ante-bellum South through an examination of plantation records. Observes that extreme care was given to pregnant mothers and their newborn infants because there was nothing more important than the increase of the slave count through the birth and rearing of children. Plantation owners took the time and effort to promote conditions that were conducive to the rearing of large families. The mortality rates of slave infants were sometimes even lower than the average in other parts of the nation for whites. Special attention was given during the term of the pregnancy, for the birth itself, and through the ante-natal years of the young.

565. Postell, W. D. "Mental Health Among Slave Populations in Southern Plantations," _American Journal of Psychiatry_ 110 (July 1953): 52-55.

Observes that the first U.S. Census Report of 1840 showed ratio of "insane" blacks to the total black population in the South to be inordinately low when compared to ratios for Northern blacks and Southern whites: (1) Southern blacks - 1 "insane" to 1400 individuals; (2) Southern Whites - 1 "insane" to 945 individuals; and (3) Northern Blacks - 1 "insane" to 144 individuals. Concludes that 1840 census was inaccurate because slave owners failed to report "insane" slaves in census because they were often able to train "deranged" slaves to perform simple, routine tasks in order to keep them working.

566. Postell, W. D. _The Health of Slaves on Southern Plantations_ (Baton Rouge: Louisiana State University Press, 1951).

The purpose of the book is to present the regime adopted by the Southern planter in caring for the health of slaves. First points out the state of the public health existing during the plantation era in the South, followed by a brief discussion of the social and economic conditions prevailing in the South. An investigation was then carried out in the various phases of plantation management that related to the health of the slaves. An attempt was made to collect and examine all data that was related to the health standards of the slaves under the topics of caring for the slaves' physical needs, the means employed in caring for those suffering from physical or mental disorders, and a description of the various diseases and injuries. The final discussion is on the analyzation and evaluation of these data from the actual results obtained in caring for the slaves. Actual results were measured in terms of death rates as compiled from the manuscript census reports and birth rates, infant mortality rates, and morbidity rates as compiled from planters' record.

567. Quiring, Daniel P. "West Indian and New Orleans Negro Metabolism Tests," Journal of Nutrition 45 (3) (November 10, 1951):443-449.

A study of metabolism of West Indians and black New Orleaneans. Begins with a discussion of the prevalence of inbreeding among the West Indians and the apparent absence of inbreeding from the Delta blacks selected. The diets of each group are discussed with some similarities in terms of fish, bread and coffee or tea. Hypertension is prevalent in the West Indian population because of the methods of food preparation, particularly salt cod. The test results show marked similarities between the two groups (height, weight and blood pressure) even though both groups lived under different economic conditions and that the metabolic rates of the two groups fell within the limits established as normal for a white population.

568. Raines, Taft. "Barriers to Community Health," Modern Hospital 79 (August 1952):71-73.

Before 1910, medical care provided to sick people in the U.S. was at a low ebb. As a result, the Carnegie Foundation sponsored a study of medical education which became known as the Flexner Report. When it was published, medical training and practice were revolutionized. One recommendation suggested by the report was for hospitals to provide access to black physicians on an equal basis as whites. Hospitals only for black physicians were not recommended. Another sweeping recommendation was that public funds not be spent on institutions which practice discrimination and that Blue Cross not approve hospitals which practice discrimination.

569. Ravitz, Mel J. "Integration of Nurses: A Latent Function of Hospital Discrimination," Phylon 16 (September 1955): 295-301.

The author attempts to explain a functional relationship between the practice of hospital discrimination among

black nurses and the integration of the nursing staff at
these hospitals, and a necessary relationship between
the practice of discrimination by the hospitals and the
socio-cultural anti-black pattern. Suggests that a
latent function of hospital discrimination is to
integrate the nursing unit at the particular hospital by
characterizing the profession as a highly selective
occupation, which screens its personnel carefully, and
bars those deemed inferior by society-at-large's values.

570. Richards, T. W. "Graduate Education of Negro
Psychologists," American Psychologist (July 1956): 326-328.

"Council on Psychological Resources in the South" became
concerned about the lack of black psychologists in the
South and therefore commissioned research of the
problem. Reports survey findings from 57 graduate
programs in Psychology in the U.S. as to the names of
black students receiving graduate degrees in psychology
and the schools from which each received their
undergraduate degrees. Found that many of the
responding universities indicated that while they would
be happy to consider admitting qualified blacks, few
black applicants were academically qualified. Concludes
that black personnel in psychology come in considerable
numbers (1/3) from black undergraduate colleges in the
South; black applicants for Ph.D. have difficulty in
meeting academic standards of graduate departments; and
Howard University is making an exceptional contribution
in providing undergraduate and masters level education.

571. Ripley, Herbert S. and Wolf, Stewart. "Studies in
Psychopathology Data Concerning Adaptation to the Isolated
Situation of a Combat Zone in the Southwest Pacific," Journal
of Nervous and Mental Disease 114 (July-December 1951):
234-250.

The authors observe that among black troops of the World
War II from a study conducted on Goodenough and Biak
Islands, blacks displayed a higher incidence of
psychoneurosis and psychosis than did the white troops.
Rigid military discipline, long working hours, and
meager facilities for entertainment enhanced the already
existing feelings among black troops of maltreatment and
racial discrimination. The authors note that black
troops' inability to easily adjust to combat conditions,
and, therefore, they suffered from a higher incidence of
mental illness. An environment of boredom, little
recreation, tropical heat, dampness, and tropical
diseases seemed to be more oppressive to black troops.

572. Rivers, Eunice, Schuman, Stanley, Simpson, Lloyd, and
Olansky, Sidney. "Twenty Years of Followup Experience in a
Long-Range Medical Study," Public Health Reports 68 (4)
(April 1953):391-395.

Discusses the non-medical aspects of the Tuskegee study.
The most important phase of the study was to follow as
many patients to death as possible in order to determine

the severity of the disease. Cooperation in this phase
was obtained by the offering of free burial assistance.
The experience of this project was beneficial as
guidance for further long-term studies. Some points
included, being aware of incentives that would produce
maximum cooperation, keep stong rapport between patient
and physician, and awareness that changes in key
personnel could have on the entire project. Also,
teamwork between all research staff members is essential
to the success to the project.

573. Rodnan, Gerald P. and Golomb, Milton W. "Gout in the
Negro Female," The American Journal of the Medical Sciences
236 (8) (September 1958): 269-283.

Reports the clinical and pathological findings of gout
in a group of six black women. In four of the cases,
the diagnosis of gout was confirmed by tophaceous
deposits in synovial biopsies or subcutaneous nodules,
or both. The other two cases were warranted on clinical
grounds despite the absence of detectable urate
collections. Renal disease was present in all the
patients. Concludes by noting that no estimate
concerning the incidence of gout within black females
can be drawn from such a small representative sample.
However, points out that the disease is more common in
black women than assumed in the past.

574. St. Clair, Harvey R. "Psychiatric Interview
Experiences With Negroes," American Journal of Psychiatry 108
(1951-52):113-119.

Addresses the need for more attention to details
observed during clinical contacts (individual) with
psychiatric patients. Argues that psychotherapy is not
different among black patients than with white with
respect to general principles and techniques, but the
above mentioned factors do carry special significance.

575. Schermerhorn, R. A. "Psychiatric Disorders Among
Negroes: A Significant Note," American Journal of Psychiatry
112 (January-June 1956):878-881.

Addresses the need for new research to give some idea of
the changing trends in psychiatric disorders among
blacks.

576. Schermerhorn, R. A. "Psychiatric Disorders Among
Negroes: A Sociological Note," American Journal of Psychiatry
(May 1956):878-882.

Argues that previous research has erroneously concluded
that the data on the differential incidences of mental
disorders among blacks and whites have been due to
inherent or ineradicable racial factors. However, many
of the disorders are truly from blacks being lower
class, the result of the strain of continuous employment
under difficult conditions, and the fact that black
children are made to feel inferior to white children.

Concludes that full scale comparison of black and white
mental patients is not possible because federal data
take no account of race.

577.   Scott, R. B., Ferguson, A. D., Jenkins, M. E., and
Cutter, F. F. "Growth and Development of Negro Infants: V.
Neuromuscular Patterns of Behavior During the First Year of
Life," Pediatrics 16 (1) (1955):24-29.

A study to determine the time of occurrence of certain
neuromuscular patterns of black infants in the first
year of life. The study sought to parallel a similar
investigation of 215 white infants through 12 behavior
steps. The steps included: smile, vocal, head control,
hand control, roll, sit, crawl, prehension, pull up,
walk with support, stand alone, walk alone. Infants
from a black clinic (a city well baby clinic) and from a
private pediatric practice are compared with the white
infants. The authors provide specific developmental
ages for the acquisition of each behavior stage for all
three groups. General findings include black infants
from the city clinic (lower socioeconomic group) showed
acceleration over black infants from private practice
from the 8th to the 35th week of life, after which, the
two groups were essentially the same. Black infants as
a whole are accelerated in their development as compared
to the white infants. Similarity was noted in the white
infants and black infants from private practice during
the first 30 weeks of life. Differences and
similarities are noted in the neuromuscular behavior and
are attributed to environmental factors. The
acceleration of black infants is a result of greater
premissiveness in child care as practiced by the mothers
or mother substitutes in the lower socioeconomic
classes.

578.   "Segregation Causes Negro Mental Illness," Science News
Letter 72 (August 3, 1957):79.

Points out that blacks in Virginia suffer from a greatly
increased rate of mental illness because of segregation
and the uncertainty accompanying cultural change. The
black rate of first admissions to the state hospitals in
proportion to black population is increasing and is now
more than double the white rate.

579.   Shafer, J. K., Usilton, Lida J., and Gleeson, Geraldine
A. "Untreated Syphilis in the Male Negro," Public Health
Reports 69(7) (July 1954):684-690.

A discussion of the disease syphilis, a disease which
exists in its acute stage for about 2 years, but the
chronicity could presist for life. The most detrimental
effects of syphilis usually occur during the first 15-20
years of the chronic period. Various other studies
about untreated syphilis were discussed along with the
methodology used. Concludes that mortality is higher
among the syphilitic individuals between the ages of 25
and 74 years of age and the life expectancy of a

syphilitic individual between 25 and 50 is about .7 percent less than the average for a non-syphilitic individual.

580. Silverstein, C. M. and Mikchell, G.   "Tuberous Sclerosis: Report of a Case with Unusual Pulmonary Manifestations," American Journal of Medicine 16 (5) (May 1954): 764-768.

A case with unusual pulmonary manifestations in a twenty-five year old colored maid, M. H. is reported. She entered the Grady Memorial Hospital on September 24, 1951, complaining of dyspnea associated with right-sided chest pain and cough. In this particular patient, asymptomatic "miliary" lesions in the lung of three years' known duration were followed by recurrent spontaneous pneumothorax and death within one year. The case is worthy of reporting because neuropsychiatric symptoms were absent and involvement of the respiratory system was the most striking clinical finding. It is suggested that other evidence of tuberous sclerosis or other malformations be searched for in patients who present themselves with spontaneous pneumothorax and cystic or "miliary" lung disease.

581.   Smith, J. L. and Merrill, I. L.   "Hereditary Hemorrhagic Telangiectasia: Nine Cases in One Negro Family, with Special Reference to Hepatic Lesions," American Journal of Medicine 17 (10) (July 1954): 41-49.

Nine cases of hereditary hemorrhagic telangiectasia in one black family and one additional autopsied case of telangiectasia of the liver are reported. Because of the rarity of reported cases of this disease in Blacks, these cases cause much attention. The difficulty in diagnosing this disease in infants is stressed. The necessity for nasopharyngoscopic examination in such cases is emphasized. Thrombocytomegaly with moderate thrombocytopenia was present in four members of this family but absent in the others. Deafness of moderate to severe degree occurred in four of ten members. Hepatomegaly occurs frequently in hereditary hemorrhagic telangiectasia. It may be due to telangiectases in the liver, posthepatitic cirrhosis, congestive heart failure secondary to anemia and the development of Laennec's cirrhosis upon exposure to alcoholism or nutritional inadequacies.

582. Spivey, O. S., Grulee, C. G. and Hickman, B. T. "Infant Tetanus Neonatorum," Journal of Pediatrics 42 (1953): 345-351.

A discussion of the occurence and prevalence of tetanus neonatorum also known as infection of the umbilical stump. Conditions for growth of various infectious organisms which cause the condition are reviewed. The problem is stated to occur in blacks four times as often as among whites. The overall high number of cases was attributed to the widespread practice of placing dung or

soot in the umbilical stump by midwives. The discussion
also includes a point of relevance as to the
socioeconomic implications of the large percentage of
infected blacks. Suggests a plan of treatment of the
infection.

583. Tucker, H. St. George, Jr., Taliaferro, Isabel,
Kirkland, Richard H. and Irby, Robert. "Addison's Disease in
the Negro," The American Journal of Medical Sciences 223 (5)
(May 1952): 479-486.

Earlier research on the topic of Addison's disease in
blacks indicated it is a rare occurrence. Presents six
cases of Addison's disease in blacks. Five of the
subjects were diagnosed clinically and one by autopsy.
Also presents data which indicates that Addison's
disease is as common among negroes as in the white
population. The pigmentary changes unique to blacks
with Addison's disease is also discussed.

584. Valien, Preston and Vaughn, Ruth E. "Birth Control
Attitudes and Practices Among Negro Mothers," Sociology and
Social Research 35 (July 1951): 415-421.

Notes that fertility rates of whites and blacks are
virtually the same in urban areas but differ in rural
areas. Observes that there are wide divergences in the
extent to which birth control is accepted and practiced.
Discusses a random sample of 100 black mothers under the
age of 40 in Nashville, Tennessee, as to their attitudes
toward birth control and birth control practices with
respect to the educational level attained by the mother,
and whether or not she was employed.

585. Wasserburger, Richard H. "Observations on the
"Juvenile Pattern" of Adult Negro Males," American Journal of
Medicine 18 (3) (March 1955): 428-437.

The unipolar electrocardiograms of 681 consecutive
admissions to the Veterans Administration Hospital,
Madison, Wisconsin, were studied for the incidence of
the "juvenile pattern." Of the total of 131 adult black
males, fourteen (10.8%) were found to show persistent or
transient T wave inversion patterns in the unipolar
leads V_1 through V_6. All fourteen patients were thought
to have normal cardiovascular systems, with no clinical
evidence of pericarditis. The "juvenile pattern" is
believed to represent an expression of hypervagotonia
and is considered to be a normal variant of the adult
Black. The author suggests that caution must be made of
these transient electrocardiogram changes in the adult
black if one wishes to avoid erroneous diagnoses of
"subepicardial myocarditis," "myocardial ischemia" and
"subacute pericarditis," and the risk of promoting
serious iatrogenic heart disease.

586. Weiss, William and Stecher, William. "Tuberculosis and
the Sickle-Cell Trait," Archives of Internal Medicine 89
(1952): 914-922.

Tuberculosis (TB) in the black race differs from that in the white race. Racial resistance to the disease must be important in determining the type of TB which develops in blacks. Studies were conducted with blacks having sicklemia (the trait) and sickled-cell (the disease). Two studies of the trait were conducted with conflicting opinions. The one at Sea View Hospital, a municipal sanitorium in New York tested 77 blacks with TB finding a 5.2 percent incidence of the trait. Philadelphia's General Hospital found a higher percentage. Herrara Cobral concludes that the frequent presence of sickled cells in the blood was the main factor in the type of TB which tends to develop in blacks. Given a case of exudative TB in a black there are 22 chances in 100 that the patient has sickling trait, twice as frequent among those having the trait. Because of the pointed shape of the red cells blood flow may be obstructed through the capillaries at least at the aerterial end of the vessel. As a result of lowered tissue resistance, the initial TB especially exudative TB, may progress and give rise to higher incidence. The sickling trait has definite clinical significance and is a factor in the response of some blacks to TB infection.

587. Wessely, Zelma. "Malignant Melanoma of Conjunctiva of the Eye of Negro Patient," A.M.A. Archives of Opthamology 62 (October 1959):697-701.

Notes the uncommon occurrence of a malignant melanoma in the eyes of American blacks. Describes a 68 year old black man admitted in 1958 to Queens General Hospital with a small, pigmented module on the bulbar conjunctiva at the limbus, a condition first noticed by the patient's optometrist six weeks prior to the patient's admission into the hospital. The patient had a past history of hypertension as well as a cholecystectomy in 1956. A physical examination of the patient's eyes led to diagnosis of malignant melanoma. Notes the failure of the tumor to pick up a significant amount of radioactive phosphorus. The left eye was thus enuclerated, and the patient was subsequently discharged.

588. Whitington, Gene L. "Congenital Nonhemolytic Icterus with Damage to the Central Nervous System: Report of a Case in a Negro Child," Pediatrics 25 (3) (March 1960): 437-440.

A case of nonhemolytic icterus with damage to the central nervous system, without familial incidence, occurring in a 2 year old black female is discussed. Jaundice began in this patient at an early age, and has been associated with severe central nervous system damage. There has been a continuous marked elevation of the indirect-reacting bilirubin in the serum. The liver is histologically normal, and neither hemolytic disorder nor biliary obstruction had been demonstrated. The fecal excretion of urobilinogen is normal. The possible relationship of this syndrome to the advances in the knowledge of bilirubin metabolism is cited.

589. Wilson, David C. et al. "The Effect of Culture Change on the Negro Race in Virginia, as Indicated by a Study of State Hospital Admissions," American Journal of Psychiatry 114 (July 1957):25-32.

Compares mental hospital data from 1914 to 1955 for whites and blacks in Virginia to determine if there was any evidence in the state hospital population to substantiate the claim that segregation causes mental illness. The data indicate that the black ratio in mental hospitals has always been higher than whites. While the white ratio increased by 113 points, the black ratio increased by 343.6. The ratio per 100,000 black population has more than doubled in forty years. Most blacks are admitted for senile psychosis, arteriosclerotic dementia, or schizophrenia.

590. Wright, Louis T. "Report from New York," The Modern Hospital 79 (2) (August 1952): 70-71.

Discusses how Harlem Hospital in New York represents an example of non-biased health care. The patients who utilize the hospital are mostly indigent with no means to attend any other hospital facility. The interesting point of the article is the fact that the staff was also operating in a non-biased fashion, Whites and blacks working together to heal whites and blacks alike. Although this hospital represented a largely indigent patient load, it also represented a goal for other hospitals to reach. The author continues a widely held belief that blacks are going to become more widely prominent in the health care field. It is stated that hopefully by the turn of the decade (1960) a real positive impact of blacks in the health care industry would be felt.

591. Young, M. D., Eyeles, D. E., Burgess, R. W. and Jeffrey, G. M. "Experimental Testing of the Immunity of Negroes to Plasmodium Vivax," The Journal of Parasitology 41 (1955): 315-318.

This report stems from the apparent inability of strains of Plasmodium Vivax to infect blacks. Experiments were set up to discover if the immunity of blacks could be overcome by massive inoculations of malaria parasites which would explain earlier published reports. Neurosyphilitic patients (mostly civilians, but including military personnel) requiring malaria therapy were inoculated either by the bites of infected mosquitos or by the injection of infected blood. The report indicates that some men were exposed daily to bites from the infected mosquitos. Among the conclusions was the following: "massive dosages of parasites, given by blood inoculation or by the bites of mosquitos, failed to overcome the immunity shown by most Negroes."

592.   Young, Martin D.   "Gongylonema Infection in South
Carolina," Journal of the American Medical Association 151
(10) (January 3, 1956): 40-41.

     A case of a black woman, 26 years of age, living in
     South Carolina who contracted Gongylonema infection.   It
     was found in the mucosa of the patient.   The probable
     cause of the infection resulted because of contamination
     by an intermediate vector.   The first reported case of a
     human infection by parasite.   Discusses the specifics of
     the condition brought about by the infection.

SUBJECT INDEX

Numbers in Subject and Author Indexes refer to entry numbers, not page numbers.

AUTHOR INDEX

A

Aaron, S.   221
Abel, J. J.   001
Abbott, G.   066, 067
Adams, N. P. G.   068
Adams, W. A.   069
Aery, W. A.   070
Afflect, T.   002
Alexander, V.   071
Allen, E. H.   073
Allen, F. P.   074
Allen, L. C.   003
Altschul, A.   075, 333
Anderson, D.   548
Anderson, G.   504
Anderson, P. F.   080, 081
Atchison, C. O.   471
Augustine, D. L.   404
Austin, B. F.   083

B

Baird, R. L.   528
Baker, B. M.   084
Bakwin, H.   085-087
Bakwin, R. M.   086
Banks, L. O.   472
Barber, J. M.   006
Barrier, J. M.   007
Bartfield, H.   473
Bartholomew, R. A.   088
Barton, R. L.   172
Bass, D. E.   474
Bauer, T. J.   172
Beck, S. J.   089
Beckham, A. S.   090
Beddoe, H. L.   475
Beeson, P. B.   259
Bender, L.   091-092
Benjamin, E. A.   093

Bennett, H. D.   476
Bent, M. J.   094-096
Berman, L. B.   477
Berstein, A.   561
Bevis, W. M.   098
Bird, R. M.   496
Black, B. K.   282
Blackman, N.   099
Blanton, W. B.   100
Blassingille, B.   478
Bloch, R. G.   101
Blount, G. W.   102
Boas, E. P.   008, 103
Boas, F.   009
Boland, F. K.   104
Bousfield, M. O.   105-108
Bowcock, H. M.   109
Boyles, P. W.   479
Brailey, M. E.   110
Branche, G. C.   111
Breidenbach, Jr. W. C   112
Brenman, M.   113
Brinton, H. P.   114
Brittain, R. H.   115-116
Brodie, J. B.   117
Brookins, S.   291
Brown, R. C.   118-120
Brown, W. R.   121
Brunner, W. F.   010
Bruyere, M. C.   181
Bruyere, P. T.   255
Bryant, B.   122
Bryant, J. E.   101
Bullock, W. H.   480
Bundesen, H. H.   172
Burch, G.   124, 378, 481, 540
Burgess, R. W.   591
Burney, L. E.   125
Burr, C. W.   011
Buskirk, E. R.   474
Butterworth, J. B.   126

ABOUT THE COMPILERS

MITCHELL F. RICE is Professor of Public Administration and Political Science at Louisiana State University, Baton Rouge. He has written extensively on Black and minority health issues in *Social Science and Medicine, Health Policy, Journal of Health and Human Resources Administration, American Journal of Preventive Medicine, Urban League Review* and other journals. He is coeditor of *Health Care Issues in Black America* (Greenwood Press, 1987) and *Contemporary Public Policy Perspectives and Black Americans* (Greenwood Press, 1984), and co-compiler of *Black American Health: An Annotated Bibliography* (Greenwood Press, 1987).

WOODROW JONES, JR. is Professor of Political Science at Texas A & M University. His writings on the topic of Black health have appeared in *American Journal of Preventive Medicine, Evaluation and the Health Profession, Urban League Review, Health Policy, Journal of Health and Human Resources Administration* and others. He is co-editor of *Contemporary Public Policy Perspectives and Black Americans* (Greenwood Press, 1984), *Health Care Issues in Black America* (Greenwood Press, 1987), and co-compiler of *Black American Health: An Annotated Bibliography* (Greenwood Press, 1987).